Natural Remedies For

Goat Diseases

Mark Gilberd
Homoeopath. Medical Herbalist and Iridologist

Index

Herbal Supplement

Herbal

Agrimony, Alfalfa, Angelica, Aniseed, Arnica, Astragalus, Barberry, Bear Berry, Black Cohosh, Blue Flag, Boswella, Broom, Burdock, Buchu, Cayenne, Calendula, Cat Mint, Cats Claw, Celery Seed, Centaury, Chamomile, Chaparral, Chaste Tree, Chickweed, Cleavers, Coltsfoot, Comfrey, Corn Silk, Cranesbill, Cranberry, Dandelion, Devils Claw, Dong Quai, Echinacea, Elecampane, Elder, Eyebright, Fennel,

Fenugreek, Feverfew, Figwort, Fumitory, Garlic, Guaiacum, Gentian, Ginger, Gingko Biloba, Ginseng Panax, Ginseng Siberian, Goldenrod, Gravel Root, Grindelia, Hawthorn, Hops, Horehound, Horse Chestnut, Horseradish, Horsetail, Hypericum, Hyssop, Juniper, Kelp, Ladys Mantle, Lemon Balm, Licorice, Lime Blossom, Marshmallow, Meadowsweet, Mistletoe, Milk Thistle, Motherwort, Mullein, Myrrh, Nasturtium, Neem, Nettles, Oats, Parsley, Passion, Flower, PauD'arco, Pennyroyal Plantain, Peppermint, Poke Root, Raspberry, Red Clover Reshi, Rose Hips, Rosemary, Rue Sage, Sarsaparilla, Shitake, Slippery Elm Bark, Shepherds Purse, Skullcap, St Johns Wort, Sweet Violets, Senna Pods, Tansy, Tea Tree Oil, Thyme, Valerian, Vervain, Wild Yam, Willow Bark, Witch Hazel, Withania Wood Betony, Wormwood, Yarrow, Yellow Dock. Yucca

Homoeopathic Suppplement

Symptoms Guide

Disease Nosodes

Materia Medica

Aconite, Allium Cepa, Ant Tart, Apis, Arnica, Arsenic Album, Belladonna, Bellis Perinnis, Bryonia, Calendula, Cantharis, Carbo Vegetabilis, Causticum, Euphrasia, Hypericum, Ipecac, Kali Bich, Kali Carb, Lachesis, Ledum, Lycopodium, Nat Sulf, Nux Vom, Phosphorus, Pulsatilla, Rhus Tox, Ruta, Silica, Staphysagria, Symphytum, Tarantula Cuba, Urtica Urens.

Vitamin C

The Safest Essential Oils For Animal Use

How Oils Work

Oils For Dogs

How Oils Work
The Golden Rules
Shampoo Formula
Oil Blends _ Formulas
Oils For Horses
The Essentials Below Are Fairly Safe For Animal Use

Introduction
Welcome To The Animal Natural Remedy Series

These books are an effort to preserve the documentation of Natural Remedies used in the treatment of animals. In the past 100 years most of these treatments have been lost, especially in the treatment of cattle one of our most ancient of farm animals. Other reasons for writing these books is that I hate vet bills and people having to kill their farm animals or pets for economic reasons which I myself have been forced to do in the past on a Goat farm. Originally these books were put together as a field reference for me for there is nothing worse than being in a paddock with a sick animal with the farmer, his hands on his hips waiting for you to perform and fix his animal.

Now the books have evolved and have had about 15 years of additions and are offered to you to teach you a new way of thinking. The books have evolved more by my different trainings. As a farmer I learnt to supplement the animals with the deficiencies of the soil so the books always start with the vitamins and minerals and their deficiency symptoms. As an Iridologist I tend to think and work with Body Systems such as The Nervous System or The Digestive System and concentrate on building them up with Nutrition and Herbs. As a Medical Herbalist I am trained to think holistically and design formulas that cover the whole being along with making the formulas easily absorbed. My Homoeopathic training teaches me to pay attention to the mind symptoms and to pay attention to what is really there not what I think is there and to treat and relieve the symptoms of the individual. Homoeopathy also shows how disease taints can be inherited and what to look for and how to treat them but best of all it gives me a special weapon to use when disaster strikes in the form of epidemics, these are called Disease Nosodes which are a preparation made from the disease product so you have a tool to help prevent the spread of disease. The books are set out in such a way as to teach you the correct use of Herbs e.g. thinking in body systems such as the Respiratory System or the Nervous System and in using herbs by their Medical Actions rather then that herb worked well last time. At the end of each system for example The Nervous System we have a section that gives you the common Actions used and needed for that section. Keeping with our example The Nervous System some of our Actions would be Anti-spasmodic, Sedative and Nervine Stimulants. After the explanation of the Action you have a list of herbs that are known to be strong in that action, this gives you more of a selection of herbs then what is mentioned in the text. Next we move on to the Homoeopathic Remedies for the condition which have the details to allow you to select a reasonably similar remedy. Homeopathy sits on a three legged stool. What this means is that if a remedy has at least three symptoms in the same strength as the symptoms you are trying to match then that remedy is a potential cure for your patient or if not cure it will offer the condition relief. The more symptoms you can match to the remedy the better the remedy will work for the rule is likes cure likes not vaguely similar cures. Homoeopathy (homo means same pathy means disease) is a good form of treatment for animals who usually respond to it fairly well and also it is very cheap to use and very easy to medicate unlike the herbs. A lot of effort has been put into the symptom details of the disease as it is very hard trying to diagnose when the animal can't answer your questions, so here you have to be very observant.

If used correctly this book makes you think and act more like a Professional Herbalist and broadens your view on what you are doing. With the Homoeopathics I have only really given you the leading remedies to put you on the right track, it would be worthwhile to invest in a good Materia Medica (Homoeopathic Remedy Reference) such as Boericke's which is one of the best for the Layman.

Main Reference Sources

The original base of the herbs I use were sourced from Juliette de Baïracli Levy's old Herbals, as hers are about the only Animal Herb References that have not been lost in time and they give you a lot of the old ancient herbs that have been used throughout most of history. To these I have added a lot of the more modern Herbs especially those that I use in my own work such as Astragalus and those that will soon be added after using for the first time on animals because there are just no substitutes. A good and recent example is Brahmi which I used in a cat recovering from a stroke because of my previous success in humans with this herb as it is supposed to rewire the brain around the damaged area and in its 3000 years of constant use someone must have used it on an Animal before. There are new herbs coming mainly from the Philippines, Indonesia, India and China but they are still being tried and tested and the average person wouldn't be able to get hold of them but the future looks far brighter than what it was 15 years ago when I started slowly putting this all together. We owe a lot to Juliette de Baïracli Levy for without her all these valuable herbs and how they were used would be lost. She has created a strong foundation that we can now build on.

Juliette de Baïracli Levy (11 November 1912 – 28 May 2009) was an English herbalist and author noted for her pioneering work in holistic veterinary medicine. Born to a wealthy Jewish family (her father was Turkish, her mother Egyptian) and raised in England with chauffeurs, maids, cooks, and gardeners. She knew as a child that she wanted to be a veterinarian. After studying veterinary medicine at the Universities of Manchester and Liverpool for two years she left England to study herbal medicine in Europe, Turkey, North Africa, Israel and Greece, living with gypsies, farmers and livestock breeders and recording their knowledge, especially the Gypsies. "I realized that if I wanted to learn the traditional ways of healing and caring for animals, I had to be where people still lived close to the land and close to their flocks," she says. "From Berbers, Bedouins, nomads, peasants, and gypsies in England, Israel, Greece, Turkey, Mexico, and Austria, I learned herbal knowledge and the simple laws of health and happiness. I never tired of traveling with my Afghan Hounds, always living with and learning from those around me." After living for some time on the Greek island Kythira she then resided in an old age home in Burgdorf, Switzerland leaving the world a better place.

For Homoeopathy my main hero is George Macleod not only for the success had based on his work but in my opinion he is a Homoeopathic Master up there with the greats and I admire his work in the use of Homoeopathic Disease Nosodes. All the high potencies mentioned are his work along with most of the Nosodes for as any trained Homoeopath knows and has had beaten into them during training you don't change the work of the masters. Unfortunately in our fast paced world not many people have time for Homoeopathy but I will say this, in the next Global Pandemic I and my family will be safe because I will make the Disease Nosode of it for I was trained by the Homoeopathic Masters.

George MacLeod (McLeod) (1912 – 1995) MRCVS DVSM Veterinary FF. Hom was a homeopathic vet, President of The British Association of Homeopathic Vets, Veterinary Consultant to The Homeopathic Development Foundation. George MacLeod was a graduate of Glasgow University and was one of the world's foremost authorities on Homeopathic treatment of animals. He was one of the few veterinary surgeons to use Homeopathic medicines wholly and exclusively. He was responsible for keeping Homeopathy available for animals in the UK, almost single-handedly, for the middle part of the 20th Century.

Other animal Homoeopaths sourced are Christopher Day, Edward Ruddock, and John Rush

Animal Natural Remedy Books

Natural Remedies For Cat Diseases
Natural Remedies For Dog Diseases
Natural Remedies For Goat Diseases
Natural Remedies For Sheep Diseases
Natural Remedies For Pig Diseases
Natural Remedies For Cow Diseases
Natural Remedies For Horse Diseases
Natural Remedies For Poultry Diseases

Mark Gilberd, Homoeopath, Iridologist, Medical Herbalist
Accredited With The Australian Traditional Medicine Society

Vitamins And Minerals

Calcium

Function - Required for the Nervous (transmission of nerve signals) and Muscular systems. Assists in the contraction of muscles. Required for blood clotting. Assists in the production of hormones and enzymes. Works with phosphorus and Vitamin D to produce bone which is 35 percent calcium. 99% of calcium in the body can be found in the bones and teeth. The absorption and maintenance of Calcium is controlled by the parathyroid gland which in turn influences the utilization of vitamin D. Calcium must always be considered in conjunction with magnesium as the two minerals interact and should be kept in balance at all times an excess of one will cause a depletion of the other. Calcium also promotes the healing of wounds and reduces acidity as well as safe guarding the health of the embryo. Dolomite contains both of these minerals. Assimilation depends on adequate amounts of Boron and Vitamins A and D in the diet.

Deficiencies - Most deficiencies are due to mineral imbalances affecting absorption. Rickets in young which leads to the deposition of uncalcified bone around the joints and bending of the long bones. In the adult animal this deficiency is called osteomalacia in which normal bone is absorbed. Developmental Orthopaedic Disease, Poor muscle function, Impaired blood clotting, Joint problems and bone weakness, Arthritis, Uneven bone growth, Knock knees, Poor teeth and lactation problems such as Milk fever, Mastitis and low milk production.

Excess - Depletes magnesium. May lead to lack of zinc uptake.

Sources - Green leafy forage, Limestone, Calcium Gluconate, Dicalcium Phosphate, Dolomite.

Herb Sources - Alfalfa, Blue Cohosh, Chamomile, Cleavers, Coltsfoot, Cayenne, Comfrey, Dandelion, Horsetail, Kelp, Mistletoe, Meadowsweet, Nettles, Parsley, Plantain, Raspberry, Rose Hips, Shepherds Purse, Yarrow, Yellow Dock.

Cobalt (Pat Coleby)

Function - Needed for healthy bone development and for the health of red blood cells, synthesised into Vitamin B12 in the gut (see B12)

Deficiencies - Cobalt anemia can cause persistent ill thrift, depleted appetite and susceptibility to cold, below normal temperature, lack of bone growth, can cause low levels of B12

Sources - Seaweed products

Copper

Function - Essential in the formation of hemoglobin as it assists in the absorption of iron, needed in the formation of cartilage and bone. Required for the correct utilization of iron in the body. Tones the nerves and helps clears septic conditions of the tissues and strengthens and brightens the hair. Copper is particularly concentrated in the liver which is the main copper storage organ. Dark skinned and dark haired animals require at least 4 times as much copper as light skinned and haired ones do.

Deficiencies - Anemia, Brittle weak bones, Faded dull coat. Possible fungal infection and internal parasites. Ringworm, Footrot, Footscald, Repeated scouring. Discolored coats in dark skinned animals (rusty blacks and faded browns) can show a deficiency. Occasionally stock will show the classic spectacle appearance when copper is deficient, the skin around the eyes appearing light colored and pulled away making the animal look as if they are wearing spectacles.

Sources - Grassland, Copper sulphate, Seaweed meal.

Herb Sources - Burdock, Chickweed, Chicory, Dandelion, Fennel, Garlic, Horseradish, Kelp, Parsley, Yarrow.

Note - Cases of copper poisoning should not occur if supplantation is carefully monitored and if the copper is always supplied with dolomite which appears to prevent toxicity. Too much copper kills but to less does the same thing. (Pat Coleby).

Fluorine

Function - Essential for the formation of healthy teeth and bones, help prevent tooth decay. Combines with calcium in the body and gives strength to the bones. Helps to keep the bones and body disease free and strengthens the eyes.

Deficiencies - Deficiencies are rare but overdosing can occur especially where soils are rich in this mineral and the water has been treated with it as well. Signs of overdosing are discolored, mottled teeth, poor condition and rough coat and lameness in the joints.

Sources - Pasture, Hay, Water and Limestone based supplements.

Herb Sources - Alfalfa, Beet leaves, Garlic, Water Cress.

Iodine

Function - Needed for correct functioning of the thyroid gland. Needed for the synthesis of thyroxine. Required for reproductive cycle to function correctly. This mineral is the supreme gland builder and conditioner, reducer of excess fatty tissue, safeguards the brain from toxins, removes toxic elements and promotes strong hair. Goats are believed to require 6 times the amount of Iodine then sheep do.

Deficiencies - Abnormal estrous cycle. Kids can be still born or born hairless while others may exhibit weakness and deformed joints. Overdosing can lead to enlarged thyroid glands. Cold weather increases the need for iodine. One of the signs of a Iodine deficiency is the presence of dandruff (scurf).

Sources - Kelp, Pasture and Mineral Licks

Herb Sources - Asparagus, Cleavers, Garlic, Kelp, Speedwell, Sarsaparilla.

Iron

Function - Essential for the formation of hemoglobin and red blood cells. Iron cannot be assimilated unless enough copper is present in the diet so a lot of anemia is caused by this. Iron carries the oxygen around the body and maintains disease resistance in the tissues.

Deficiencies - Anemia, Poor Performance, Poor growth in young stock.

Sources - Grasslands and Cereals.

Herb Sources - Alfalfa, Asparagus, Bilberry, Burdock, Blue Cohosh, Cayenne, Chicory, Comfrey, Dandelion, Gentian, Hawthorn, Hops, Mullein, Nettles, Parsley, Raspberry, Skullcap, Vervain, Yellow Dock.

Manganese

Function - Required for the utilization of fats and carbohydrates. Essential for the formation of cartilage, assists in the formation of bones and enzymes.

Deficiencies - Cows that become deficient can give birth to deformed calves whose bones are not correctly developed. Infertility. Deficiency is fairly rare.

Sources - Wheat Bran and Grasslands

Herb Sources - Kelp.

Magnesium

Function - Required for hemoglobin formation in the blood. Between 50 and 70% of ingested magnesium is needed for bone growth and the balance is used for neuro-muscular transmission, muscular health and a healthy nervous system. Magnesium uptake can be depressed by too much calcium (see Calcium). Assists in enzyme functions of the body and reduces excess acidity.

Deficiencies - Nervousness and excitability. Increased respiratory rates. Muscle tremors. Tetany, Aggressiveness and ill temper, mastitis, arthritis, warts, soft teeth and deformed bones.

Sources - Alfalfa, Clover, Bran, Linseed, Magnesium Carbonate and Dolomite.

Herb Sources - Alfalfa, Blue Cohosh, Broom, Carrot leaves, Cayenne, Dandelion, Hops, Marshmallow, Meadowsweet, Mistletoe, Mullein, Peppermint, Raspberry, Slippery Elm.

Molybdenum

Function - Needed for maximum fertility, co factor to a number of oxidase enzymes, involved in fat metabolism and iron and copper metabolism. Excess copper and sulphate increases demand.

Deficiencies - Asthma, dental caries, mental disturbances.

Sources - Legumes, oats, sunflower seeds, wheat germ.

Potassium

Function - Works with sodium to assist in correct nerve function and muscular contractions. Important along with others for the osmotic regulation of body fluids and in acid - base balance. Assists in maintaining the correct fluid balance in the body. Promotes general healing of the tissues, tones the bowels, gall bladder and liver.

Deficiencies - Weight loss, Diarrhea, Muscle weakness, Difficult births, anemia, scour.

Excess - Interferes with magnesium uptake.

Source - Green forage and Molasses.

Herb Sources - Alfalfa, Blue Cohosh, Borage, Carrot leaves, Chamomile, Coltsfoot, Comfrey, Couch Grass, Centaury, Dandelion, Elder, Eyebright, Fennel, Kelp, Ladies Mantle, Mistletoe, Meadowsweet, Mullein, Nettles, Parsley, Peppermint, Plantain, Raspberry, Shepherds Purse, Skullcap, Wormwood, Yarrow.

Phosphorous

Function - Essential for healthy growth and life. Works with calcium for bone growth. Vital in energy metabolism and the formation of high energy bonds with in cells. A component of the amino acids Methionine and Cystine along with phospholipids and nucleic acids. An integral component of just about every enzyme system. Builds and maintains the brain, teeth and hair. Makes up 15 percent of bone. Too much phosphorous will reduce the absorption of calcium and magnesium during digestion leading to problems.

Deficiencies - There are extensive areas of phosphorus deficient soils especially in tropical and sub-tropical areas, deficiency can be exaggerated by lack of vitamin D and may cause reduced growth rate, inefficient breeding, defects and fractures of bones and Pica (depraved appetite). Overfeeding of phosphorous can lead to lameness, fragile bones, enlargement of the jaw bone, hyperparathyroidism and maybe Botulism.

Excess - Reduces calcium and magnesium

Sources - Cereals, Grains, Bone meals, Dicalcium Phosphate, Dolomite.

Herb Sources - Alfalfa, Anise, Asparagus, Blue Cohosh, Caraway, Cayenne, Chickweed, Calamus, Dandelion, Dill, Fenugreek, Garlic, Golden Rod, Kelp, Licorice, Linseed, Marigold, Meadowsweet, Parsley, Raspberry, Rose Hips, Sunflower, Yellow Dock.

Selenium

Function - Works with Vitamin E. Essential part of antioxidant enzymes which help to remove toxins from the system. Assists in maintaining a healthy immune system. A small amount is needed for fertility and for healthy muscles and growth.

Deficiencies - In foals it can cause hair loss, loss of growth, dark urine, labored breathing and white muscle disease. Overfeeding can cause poisoning. If the kid responds to Vitamin E then it probably is short on selenium to.

Sources - Pastures, Alfalfa, Sea weed, Brewers Grains and Linseed.

Sulphur

Function - Most sulphur is in the form of sulphur containing amino acids with methionine and cystine as some examples. Some vitamins contain sulphur mainly thiamine and biotin . Assists in enzyme and hormone production. Sulphur is often beneficial for skin ailments both topically and internally. Sulphur acts as a purifier and tonic for the entire system especially the blood. Maintains health of the skin and hair, strengthens the glandula system and promotes the flow of bile and keeps the liver healthy.

Deficiencies - None recorded but overdosing can lead to loss of weight and appetite, colic, a yellow frothy discharge from the nose and laboured breathing. Goats that are sulphur deficient may have lice, ticks or other exterior parasites (Pat Coleby), Skin ailments.

Sources - Protein feeds and Green forage.

Herb Sources - Alfalfa, Burdock, Broom, Calamus, Coltsfoot, Cayenne, Daisy, Eyebright, Fennel, Garlic, kelp, Marigold, Meadowsweet, Mullein, Nettle, Parsley, Plantain, Raspberry, Sage, Shepherds purse, Thyme, Yarrow.

Sodium Chloride

Function - Maintains the balance of fluids in the cells. Assists in muscle contractions. Helps in the acid - base balance. Removes waste products from the cells. Required in the production of bile. Maintains the health of the nervous system.

Sources - Salt and salt licks. Green forages especially Alfalfa.

Deficiencies - Dehydration, Poor Growth, Muscle cramps. Over feeding of salt can result in high blood pressure.

Zinc

Function - Assists in the metabolism of nutrients. Required for the immune system to function correctly. Needed for healthy skin, hair and hooves. Necessary for a healthy reproductive system both in sexes. Assists in blood formation. May also be needed when recovery from sickness is not as fast as it should be. Is a constitute of many enzyme systems as well as a activator of such systems.

Deficiencies - Can lead to dry flaky skin, eczema, hair loss and poor growth loss.

Herb Sources - Kelp and Marshmallow.

Vitamins

Vitamin A (retinol)

Function - Helps to maintain epithelial tissues which cover the body and line certain internal organs. This vitamin is also essential for proper growth of skeletal and soft tissues especially the light sensitive areas of the eyes. Needed for hormone synthesis, bone growth, and used in most of the mucous membranes of the body. Needed for proper eye function.

Deficiencies - Night blindness, Excessive tears, Rough coat, Lack of appetite, Infections of the reproductive tract, Poor growth and weak bones and tendons, there can be infertility, colostrum can be low in vitamin A and as a result new born animals succumb to scour and pneumonia.

Sources - Carrots, Carotene in green leafy plants and Cod Liver Oil.

Herb Sources - Alfalfa, Burdock, Cayenne, Comfrey, Dandelion, Kelp, Marshmallow, Papaya, Parsley, Raspberry, Red Clover, Watercress, Yellow Dock.

B1 Thiamine

Function - Assists in metabolizing carbohydrates. Maintains a healthy nervous system. Assists in energy metabolism. Has been found to have a calming effect when fed to nervous horses. Can assist in the performance and stamina of competition horses. This vitamin is made by microflora in the intestines.

Deficiencies - Weight loss, Muscular weakness, Muscular incoordination and missed heart beats. Deficiencies are fairly rare due to this vitamin being made in the intestines but are mainly seen in young stock reared intensively on manufactured feed with little or no roughage. In humans deficiency causes Beriberi.

Sources - Good forage, Good hay, Cereal grains and Brewer's Yeast.

Herb Sources - Cayenne, Dandelion, Fenugreek, Kelp, Parsley, Raspberry.

B2 Riboflavin

Function - Maintains a healthy nervous system. Functions as a coenzyme concerned with the oxidative process. Assists in energy metabolism. This vitamin is also made in the intestines.

Deficiencies - Rough coat and dry skin, Conjunctivitis, Excessive tearing and may be connected with moon blindness. Deficiencies are fairly rare. In humans can cause open sores in the corner of the mouth and on the lips and sometimes seborrheic dermatitis.

Sources - Green forage, Good hay and milk.

Herb Sources - Alfalfa, Burdock, Fenugreek, Kelp, Parsley, Watercress.

B3 Niacin

Function - Helps in the metabolism of nutrients and also with hormone and lipid syntheses. This vitamin is also made in the intestines.

Deficiencies - None recorded. Over dosing may cause dilation of blood vessels, sickness and itching of skin. Deficiencies in humans causes Pellagra.

Sources - Green forage especially Lucerne.

Herb Sources - Alfalfa, Burdock, Fenugreek, Kelp, Parsley, Sage.

B5 Pantothenic Acid

Function - Assists in energy metabolism and the formation of anti-bodies.

Deficiencies - Deficiency is rare as this vitamin is made in the intestines.

Sources - Green forage, Cereals and Peas.

B6 Pyridoxine

Function - Assists in energy metabolism. maintains health of the nervous system. Assists in the formation of hemoglobin in the blood. Maintains the health of the immune system. Heavily worked horses have benefited from B6 supplementation. This vitamin is made in the bowel.

Deficiencies - None recorded.

Sources - Green forage and Cereal grains.

Herb Sources - Alfalfa, Chlorophyll

B12 Cyanocobalamin

Function - This vitamin contains the metal Cobalt. Assists in the production of red blood cells. Assists in energy metabolism. It is important in many enzyme systems and is necessary for the metabolism of propionic acid in the ruminant. Can assist in putting on condition and correcting anemia. This vitamin is made in the bowel. Inability to absorb this vitamin cause Pernicious Armenia.

Deficiencies - Mainly seen in young and growing animals causing retarded growth, anemia, and high mortality. Deficiencies of B12 in ruminants are largely the result of low levels of dietary Cobalt.

Sources - Green forages.

Herb Sources - Alfalfa, Chlorophyll, Dong Quai, Kelp.

Biotin

Function - Assists in the metabolism of energy. Active in enzyme systems involved with carbohydrate metabolism, fatty acid and protein synthesis and amino acid deamination. Maintains sebaceous glands in the skin. Maintains bone marrow.

Deficiencies - Maybe foot problems.

Sources - Yeast, Green forage and Cereals.

Choline

Function - Assists in the transport of fats stored in

the liver to other areas of the body for use as energy. Maintains a healthy nervous system. Is an essential structural component of body tissue with a vital role in cell structure and activity.

Deficiencies - Can lead to poor growth and increased storage of fats in the liver.

Sources - Natural Fats, Green leafy forage and Yeast cereals.

Folic Acid

Function - Assists cell metabolism. Required for red blood cell formation. Assists in general metabolism.

Deficiencies - Anemia and poor growth. Prolonged use of sulphur drugs in ruminants depress the bacterial synthesis of this vitamin.

Sources - Green leafy forage

Vitamin C (ascorbic acid)

Function - Essential for the formation of collagen tissue which is vital in tendons and cartilage. Essential for the utilization of essential amino acids lysine and proline. Needed for the transport of iron to storage organs.

Deficiencies - None recorded. Supplementation has been given in periods of stress and growth. Causes Scurvy in humans

Sources - Made in the liver and other body cells. Fresh fruits and vegetables.

Herb Sources - Alfalfa, Burdock, Catnip, Cayenne, Chickweed, Dandelion, Hawthorn, Garlic, Horseradish, Kelp, Parsley, Plantain, Papaya, Raspberry, Rosehips, Shepherds Purse, Yellow Dock.

Vitamin D

Function - Essential for the absorption of phosphorus and calcium and for growth maintenance and repair of bones and teeth, sterols are converted into vitamin D by ultra violet light, latter parts in the conversion process are controlled by the parathyroid.

Deficiencies - Can be caused by lack of exposure to the sun and may cause - Reduced growth, weak bones and increased bone problems, failure to absorb calcium and phosphorus. Rickets, Osteomalacia, Osteoporosis.

Sources - Cut and dried plants, Fish Oils and through the skin after contact with sunlight.

Herb Sources - Alfalfa, Chlorophyll, Don Quai, Kelp.

Vitamin E

Function - Helps with the immune system and is a powerful antioxidant. Helps stabilize cell membranes and acts on the reproductive system, works with selenium.

Deficiencies - Anemia, Swelling of joints, muscular incoordination and reduced stamina.

Sources - Leafy green forage, Good hay, Cereals and

Alfalfa.

Herb Sources - Alfalfa, Dandelion, Dong Quai, Kelp, Raspberry, Rose Hips, Water Cress.

Vitamin K

Function - Helps in the clotting of blood and in calcium assimilation.

Deficiencies - Bleeding and longer blood clotting time.

Sources - Made in the gut from green leafy forage.

Herb Sources - Alfalfa, Chlorophyll, Plantain, Shepherds Purse.

Digestive System

Acute Indigestion

This is usually a disturbance of function without pathological changes taking place. Overeating is a frequent cause and may relate to normal or other foods such as grains or cake etc. Damaged or spoilt food can also be a cause. In kids colic or abdominal pain is the most common symptom of indigestion. Other causes can be drenching with linseed or Cod liver oil and in these cases the rumenal contents are so unpleasant that the Goat refuses to chew the cud or will spit it out when regurgitated.

Signs and Symptoms

Acute indigestion may be accompanied by bloat. Simple cases show a lack of appetite with a slight increase in the rate of respiration. The faeces may be hard or watery depending on the nature of the food taken. Rumenal contractions are usually reduced when the dung is dry and increased when diarrhea is present. Rumenal impaction produces a doughy feeling with reduced stomach movement. Severe overloading of the rumen may lead to toxemia if treatment is not started early with recumbency, sluggish reflexes and sub normal temperature being present.

Herbal Treatment

Sometimes a good purge with Epsom Salts can be

given so as to clear out the system, then new fresh food can be introduced with some animals having to be forced feed by having the food pushed to the back of the mouth. Fresh cud from healthy animals can be mixed with water to form a drench and be used to replace normal bacterial flora. Clove tea can be used to help a Goat regain its appetite, to make put 12 cloves in 500mls of water, boil and simmer for 10 minutes and when cool divide into 3 parts and drench 3 times a day. A drench of Chamomile tea can be helpful for indigestion especially if it is accompanied by colicky pain. A Herbal Tonic for cows with poor appetite could be used here for the goat but in a reduced strength. The recipe is a level teaspoon full of Gentian Powder with a level teaspoon full of Ginger with the same amount of Caraway Seeds and Anise Seeds (crush the seeds to release the oils) along with a couple of powdered charcoal tablets all mixed in a cup and the add boiling water, stir and cover (to keep in the essential oils). Give a cup of this in the evenings. Sometimes human Quick Ease tablets can be a cure for simple indigestion.

Homoeopathic Treatment

Abies Canadensis 30C - Useful remedy when simple overeating is the cause. Abdominal flatulence arises. Dose 3 times daily for 3 days.

Carbo Veg 200C - Indicated when pronounced bloating is present accompanied by toxaemia and tendency for coma. Dose one every hour for 4 doses.

Colchicum 30C - To much green food precipitating

the condition calls for this remedy when bloat is present. The bowels are usually loose. Dose 3 times daily for 4 days.

Nux Vom 1M - Indicated when the condition arises from the eating of indigestible fodder. Constipation is usually present. Dose 3 times daily for 4 days.

Lycopodium 200C - Mild cases of bloat may benefit from this remedy. The lower right hand side of the abdomen feels full due to sluggish liver activity. Dose daily for 5 days.

Bloat

Acute tympany of the rumen is a specific form of indigestion which can arise suddenly when gas in the rumen is produced faster than it is eliminated. Bloat occurs in Goats fed on lush legumes such as Lucerne, clovers or lush spring pastures. It often occurs on a Monday morning in urban Goats as the owners frequently gather lush feed over the weekend. To help prevent Bloat always provide some dry hay or dry pasture when feeding fresh legumes.

Pat Coleby says Bloat is a sign of a sick farm with the cause being an imbalance of potassium, magnesium, sulphur and boron. He say that if the farm had been farmed organically and re-mineralized the bloat would not of happened because the stands of solid clover that so often cause Bloat only grow on unbalanced , over fertilized and under mineralized soil.

Signs and Symptoms

A fullness or swelling, small at first appears over the left sub-lumber region. This swelling increases rapidly as the rumen fills with gas. In well-marked cases the flank at its upper part rises above the level of the backbone and when struck with the tips of the fingers sounds like a drum. The Goat is very distressed, stamps its feet, bleats, urinates frequently and walks with a stilted action. Soon the swelling becomes hard and tense, while difficulty in breathing may be severe. The distension of the stomach may become so great as to prevent the animal from breathing and in some cases may be complicated by rupture of the stomach. Bloat may be frothy in type when salivation is common in addition to other symptoms. If the distension continues rapidly the goat will fall down on its side with the breathing becoming worse and if nothing is done may die in 30 minutes.

Treatment

In mild cases walking the goat around the yard and then standing her front feet on a box and massaging the swollen flank should make them belch and relieve the situation. If this fails drench with 100mls of cooking oil as oily preparations break up the gas bubbles and repeat the above again as the walking and massage will spread the oil in the rumen and may allow the gas to be passed from one end or another.

If the above procedure fails all that's left is to

puncture the rumen to let the gas out which is best left to a vet or if in a emergency done while you have the vet on the phone. A sharp pointed thin bladed knife should be sterilized and inserted (See Picture) until the gas starts to escape twist the knife slightly to encourage the release of gas then remove and close the wound.

Homoeopathic Treatment

If discovered in time the following remedies will be of some use.

Antimonium Crud 6C - Useful in frothy bloat which comes on quickly after eating. Dose every hour for 4 doses.

Apis 6C - This remedy will help control the amount of fluid generated by frothy bloat. Dose every half hour for 4 doses.

Carbo Veg 6C - This is suitable for less acute cases. The animal shows signs of impending toxaemia. Dose every hour for 4 doses.

Colchicum 6C - More acute cases if seen in time will respond to this remedy. Dose every half hour for 6 doses.

Colic

Causes can be from excess feeds of lush greens especially if new to the Goat or frosted greens, or in bad cases a foreign body or maybe poison. In kids it may be caused by violent exercise after a large feed of milk. Care should be taken when introducing animals to new pastures. Over exposure to dampness or chill winds can be another cause of colic.

Signs and Symptoms

Acute pain in the abdomen, the animal attempts to lie in a unusual position, groans, rolls and attempts to kick its belly. Sometimes the belly can be distended and there can be similar signs to bloat like a roached back and striking the ground with their feet. Some times in bad cases kids will fling themselves about as though epileptic. Also in some cases the eyes are congested. Unlike horses ruminants do not sweat when suffering from Colic spasms.

Herbal Treatment

Fast immediately and in bad cases give a laxative so as to clear the irritant out of the system with castor oil being good for this. Give a fluid diet for several days of barley meal gruel with milk, honey and Slippery Elm with crushed Chlorophyll Tablets mixed in. If pains become bad give a brew of Licorice, Chamomile and Dill seeds (About a heaped teaspoonful of each, don't forget to crush the seeds so as to release the oil) in a cup, add boiling water and mix well and then cover and leave till tepid, strain then drench. Another proven herbal drench is a strong brew of Mint and Thyme.

Homoeopathic Treatment

Aconite 6C - Always in the early stages, intense thirst, abdomen sensitive to touch, especially good if the temperature is rising , one dose every hour for 4 doses
Belladonna 1M - Full bounding pulse early in the condition, sweating, dilated pupils and excitability,

skin hot and smooth, thirst is prominent along with colicky pains. Dose every 2 hours for 4 doses.

Colchicum 6C - Distension of abdomen and rumbling of flatus, lower parts of the bowel become distended and can be felt on the right side, animal tends to remain standing, Dose every hour for 3 doses.

Colocynthis 1M - When spasmodic colic has severe pain and appears to result from having eaten green food. Motions are watery with wind, onset and relief are abrupt. Dose every 4 hours for 4 doses.

Dioscorea 6C - Unbearable sharp, cutting, twisting pain that radiates to distant parts, some relief from stretching out or bending backwards. Dose every 4 hours for 4 doses.

Mag Phos 6X - Spasms of cramp which are relieved by warmth and gentle massage. Dissolve dose in 5mls of warm water and give every 20 minutes for 4 doses.

Nux Vom 6C - If the attack was brought on by eating indigestible food or overeating. Straining to pass dung or urine, animal lies on its side looking uneasy, bending head towards flank. Dose every 2 hours for 4 doses.

Diarrhea and Dysentery (Enteritis)

Diarrhea is purging or looseness of the bowels in which the discharges are faecal. Causes in Goats can be improper food, putrid water, worms, Cobalt and Copper deficiencies, exposure to damp and cold weather and as a result of a debilitated constitution. The best cure is by removing the cause. Dysentery can follow neglected diarrhea.

Signs and Symptoms

The dung is loose and latter becomes liquid and is sometimes spurted out to a distance, there may or may not be griping pains. If the animal retains strength and appetite the diarrhea may be regarded as an effort of nature to remove some unhealthy matter and should not be stopped. Long continued and violent diarrhea must be treated.

Herbal Treatment

The best cure here is to try and remove the cause and if the condition gets worse treat as dysentery. If the problem looks serious give a laxative drench to sweep the putrid matter from the intestines. A quick effective drench is one or two ounces of Epsom Salts dissolved in a pint brew of Dill Seed water (one small handful of dill seeds boiled for 5 minutes). Senna Pods can also be used as a laxative drench. Fast the Goat for 24 hours following the drench and give garlic brew or tablets in the evening for internal disinfecting. Reintroduce food slowly with a gruel like mentioned in Indigestion but add to this Slippery Elm which will soothe and gently astringe the intestines along with adding nourishment. Pat Colbey says sometimes a desert spoon of Vitamin C and a desert spoon of dolomite along with a quarter of a teaspoon full of Copper sulphate can cure diarrhea. He says half this amount can be given to kids with scour. With worms there is usually a copper deficiency.

Dysentery is inflammation of the mucous membranes of the bowels attended with increased secretion of mucous, sometimes blood and with increased straining. This can also be part and a symptom of a more serious disease such as enterotoxaemia, Coccidiosis or some plant poisoning such as Deadly Nightshade.

Signs and Symptoms

There may be loss of spirits and appetite, slight gripping pains and frequent straining passing a quantity of wind and mucous usually mixed with blood or with shreds of mucous membrane and there may be fever.

Herbal Treatment

Treatment is similar to Diarrhea. If case is severe start off with a laxative drench. Cease all food for at least 24 hours maybe more. Slippery Elm is our main herb for Dysentery as it is mildly astringent and very demulcent and in this case mix it with lots of honey so as to encourage eating as well as making it very nutritious. To this we add about 10 garlic oil capsules which are there to disinfect the bowel along with some chlorophyll and a hand full of charcoal with these last 2 being there to cleanse and absorb the toxins and gas. As the intestines heal milk should be added to the Slippery Elm and honey gruel along with 1 small teaspoon full of Gentian to one and a half pints of gruel. When dysentery lessens the gruel diet should be broken with the feeding for several days of a warm mash of flaked barley to which a little powdered Marsh Mallow root can be added.

Note - See Emergency Rehydration Liquid (electrolytes) in Scour.

Homoeopathic Treatment

Aconite 30C- Diarrhea in the primary stage, at the beginning of acute cases that come on suddenly and violently, when it arises from taking cold, considerable fever, inflammation of the bowels, can be alternated with Nux Vom. Dose - every half hour for 4 doses.

Nux Vom 12X - Discharges slimy and offensive with rumbling noises in the bowels and passing of wind, when there are symptoms of indigestion and when purging is alternated with constipation for example frequent passing of 1 or 2 small feculent balls accompanied by tenesmus. Dose once every 2 hours.

Arsenicum 1M - For watery, slimy, greenish or brownish diarrhea, with or without gripping pains and can smell offensive, great rumbling in the bowels and flatulence, total loss of appetite and a marked prostration of strength, skin and extremities cold great restlessness. Dose - every hour for 4 doses.

China 30C - Useful in chronic cases or when caused by hot weather and not of a inflammatory character, painless discharge, loss of appetite and strength. Can be used as a tonic when acute symptoms have passed away, evacuations consist partly of undigested food, can be pain during discharge.

Bryonia 30C- If the disorder has been brought on by a change of temperature especially from hot to cold, by drinking cold water or impure water, faeces are very watery and involuntary passed and may contain undigested food, can be alternating diarrhea and constipation. Dose four times a day.

Mercurius Cor 200C- Frequent discharge of mucous tinged with blood or thin bloody and foetid stools, frequent urging to stool, redness and swollen appearance of the anus, symptoms worse at night. Dose 3 times daily for 3 days.

Colocynthis 6C - Nausea, severe colicky pains, slimy evacuations or mucous tinged with blood, distension of the bowels and pain on pressure, tenesmus, thirst, variable temperature of the body being at one time shivering and soon after very hot. Dose every half hour for 4 doses.

Chamomilla 30C If there is pain just before a evacuation which can be of a greenish color with mucous. Dose four times a day

Note - See also Coccidiosis and Enterotoxaemia in the disease section.

Scour (Indigestion and Dysentery in Kids)

The causes are fairly similar to indigestion. Other causes may be a acid and alkali imbalance, failure to ingest colostrum after birth, lack of sanitation or worms and in this case it would be worthwhile finding out the names of the worms so you can treat all the stock

Signs and Symptoms

The Kid is depressed, the appetite is poor, sometimes there is fever, the extremities may be cold along with the nose and there may be a rapid and weak pulse. The dung becomes gradually softer and lighter in color until it is cream colored and a little thicker then milk. It has a most offensive odor and may contain clumps of curd. Latter it contains mucous and gas bubbles (at this stage action must be taken quick). It sticks to the hair of the tail and buttocks causing the hair to drop off and the skin to become irritated. There may be pain on passing dung and also abdominal colicky pain. The Kid stands about with its back arched and its belly contracted. There may be tympanites. In severe cases there is sudden prostration with great weakness and without treatment will lead to death. A frequent sequel can be Pneumonia.

Herbal Treatment

Remove the cause; give the appropriate feed of best quality in small doses. If being bottle fed make sure all utensils are clean. The speediest cure for scouring bottle fed Kid is to let them suck from a healthy Goat. Treatment should begin with a laxative drench to sweep the putrid matter out of the intestines. A quick effective drench is 1 or 2 ounces of Epsom's salts dissolved in 1 and a half pints of a brew of Dill seed and water or Senna pods. (One hand full of Dill seeds brewed for 15 minutes in 1 and half pints of water.) After this fast the Kid for 24 hours and give some garlic capsules in the evening for internal disinfecting. On the second day give 3 meals of milk mixed with the same amount of water, add to this 1 teaspoon full of molasses and then the main ingredient which is slippery elm. If the Kid is not eating give some of this in a drench and see what happens. Make sure there is lots of fresh clean water especially if it is a hot day as Kids dehydrate fairly fast. Towards the end of the third day slowly introduce its normal food but very carefully. Pat Colbey says sometimes a Teaspoon of Vitamin C and a teaspoon of dolomite can cure diarrhea.

Note - Emergency Rehydration Liquid (electrolytes)
Homemade Electrolyte Solution
Since death results from dehydration and shock the first goal is to restore the electrolyte balance.
 2 tablespoons of salt
1 teaspoon of baking soda
8 tablespoons of honey
1 gallon of water.

Homoeopathic Treatment
Look at the remedies listed under Diarrhea and Dysentery especially China in long standing cases, other remedies are listed below.
Aconite 30C- Diarrhea in the primary stage, at the beginning of acute cases that come on suddenly and violently, when it arises from taking cold, considerable fever, inflammation of the bowels, can

be alternated with Nux Vom. Dose every half hour for 4 doses.

China 30C - Useful when caused by hot weather and not of a inflammatory character, painless discharge, loss of appetite and strength. Of great value in helping to restore strength after loss of body fluid. Can be used as a tonic when acute symptoms have passed away, evacuations consist partly of undigested food , can be pain during discharge.

Cuprum Aceticum 6C - A useful remedy for scouring calves, the abdomen is usually tympanic prior to evacuation, stools may be dark with blood stained mucous, animal is generally weak and trembling. Dose every 2 hours for 4 doses followed by one twice daily for 3 days.

Veratrum Album 30C - General appearance of collapse with signs of abdominal pain preceding the onset of diarrhea, stools are watery and forcibly evacuated, body sweating is present, the Goat is cold and there may be a bluish tinge to the mucous membranes. Dose every 2 hours for 4 doses.

Carbo Veg 200C - Stools are preceded by signs of abdominal colic with flatulence, it is a excellent remedy for helping revive apparently moribund patients, such Goats should be given access to fresh air. Dose every hour for 4 doses.

Dulcamara 30C - A useful remedy if the onset of disease symptoms is associated with exposure to damp, Dose 3 times daily for 2 days.

Mercurius Cor 200C- Frequent discharge of mucous tinged with blood or thin bloody and foetid stools, frequent urging to stool, redness and swollen appearance of the anus, symptoms worse at night. Dose 3 times daily for 3 days.

Constipation (Impaction)

This is not very general in Goats and occurs mostly in stall kept animals (too much concentrates) though constipation can be a symptom of another disease or health problem especially liver problems. Make sure Goat has access to lots of water.

Signs and Symptoms

Straining and passage of small hard dry lumps of dung which may be covered with slimy mucous, the breath may be foul and the eyes inflamed.

Herbal Treatment

Look to the diet so as to try and find and correct the cause as constipation is more common in stall kept animals. Give a very green and laxative diet and use the following reliable purge for several days. Mix 2 tablespoons of powdered licorice with 1 dessertspoonful of powdered Ginger and add to this 2 ounces of Castor Oil. Mix all together and make paste into round balls. Pulped carrots and parsnips and berry fruits can be added to the diet to help matters.

Pat Coleby for this condition gives 500ml drench of a good vegetable oil for a large Goat followed by a teaspoon of ascorbate (Vitamin C powder)as a drench, which also has a mild laxative effect and would restore the health of the gut. Never use liquid paraffin as it demineralizes the body and this could be dangerous for kids.

Homoeopathic Treatment

Nux Vom 6C - Uncomplicated cases, when there is ingestion of indigestible food. Dose every 2 hours for 3 doses in mild cases. In animals subject to a more chronic condition give a 1M dose night and morning for 2 days.

Sulphur 6C - Abdomen sensitive to pressure and colicky symptoms after drinking. This remedy can most usefully be employed in conjunction with Nux Vom giving the remedies in alternation.

Hydrastis 30C - General catarrhal states, signs of stiffness over lumber region, liver dysfunction and jaundice may be present. Dose 3 times daily for 3 days.

Mag Mur 6C - Liver dysfunction, yellow tongue and other signs of jaundice may appear, stools small and crumbly, Dose 3 times daily for 3 days.

Bryonia 6C - Stools large hard and may contain blood especially in young animals. Dose 3 times daily for 3 days.

Purge For Goats

A effective purge for Goats is 2 ounces of Epsoms Salts, one ounce of linseed oil, half a teaspoonful of ground ginger, one teaspoonful of grated Gentian root and 2 ounces of warm water, give mixed in oatmeal gruel to make 1 and a half pints, Kids can be given a quarter part of this laxative.

Liver Problems

Jaundice

This can occur as a symptom of inflammation of the liver or sluggish function without inflammation maybe from a congested liver. Obstruction of the bile ducts is another obvious cause. The main cause may be a unsuitable diet especially over prolonged use of concentrated unnatural cakes and meals which may of overloaded and congested the liver. Also vermifuges (wormers) may over time damage the liver and produce jaundice.

Signs and Symptoms

The mucous membranes of the eyes, mouth and nose become tinged with yellow and the skin also shows this discoloration. Urine becomes dark green because of the presence of bile, constipation may be present, faeces is light in color and in some cases there may be edema of the limbs. Pressure along the margin of the short ribs produces pain, the appetite is poor and the animal shows hardly any inclination to drink (can be the opposite to), the animal lays down much and moves with reluctance , has a tottering gait. Sometimes the animal has a dry painful cough and presents a dull stupefied appearance and there may be foul smelling breath.

Herbal Treatment

It is the derangement of the bile flow which is the basic cause for this complaint and until it is normalized the yellow pigment will continue to be noticeable especially in the eyes. Give a short fast with a non-oily purge (Senna pods , Epsom's Salts). All fatty foods should be avoided in the diet (no linseed, sunflower etc) also avoid giving pulse foods. Give a abundance of Dandelion in the diet the roots can be grated and included as well. Also recommended are Cleavers and Centaury. Otherwise the diet should be mainly grass and other leafy green vegetables, bran. Molasses, carrots and seaweed. Some other herbs to look at are Milk Thistle, Blue Flag and Speedwell.

Speedwell - Used for jaundice, impure blood, dysentery, gastric insufficiency, cough, asthma etc.

Homoeopathic Treatment

Aconite 30C - Give at the onset of the problem especially if it arises from cold or there is fever.

Berberis Vulgaris 30C - Sluggish liver conditions with tenderness over lumber region. Skin yellowish, urinary symptoms present. Dose 3 times daily for 3 days.

Chelidonium 6C - Pain and tenderness over right shoulder area. Strong yellow discoloration of visible mucous membranes. Obstruction of bile ducts. Dose 3 times daily for 3 days.

China 30C - Weakness and debility, abdominal pain, stools yellow and fluid, increasing weakness. Dose every 3 hours for 4 doses.

Lycopodium 200C - Flatulent state, indifferent appetite, abdominal tympany after eating, mucous membranes greyish yellow and urine loaded with red sediment. Dose night and morning for 5 days.

Mag Mur 30C - Enlargement of liver with difficulty in urination, jaundice and abdominal pain pronounced. Dose night and morning for 4 days.

Herbal Overview Of The Digestive System

In dealing with problems of the digestive system its always best to start with a purge so as to clean the system and bowels out. This is very important especially when you do not know what you are dealing with because you are purging out hopefully most of the toxins that are causing the condition. After the purge isolate and fast the animal for 24 hours and see what happens.

Below are a list of Herbal Actions that are used for the digestive system read through them and become familiar with them for in Herbal Medicine you always think in actions needed not the Herb needed this way the mind stays on the big picture.

Herbal Actions For The Digestive System

Anti-biotic - Always start with Garlic as this is both anti-bacterial and anti-viral as well as being used for killing parasites and worms, your initial attack begins here.

Herbs - Echinacea, Garlic, Myrrh, Pau D' Arco, Reshi.

Anti-emetic - Can reduce a feeling of nausea and can help to relieve or prevent vomiting.

Herbs - Cayenne, Fennel, Meadowsweet, Peppermint,

Anti-inflammatory - Helps the body to combat inflammations, there will always be pain, heat and maybe fever when these are called for. Herbs mentioned under demulcents will often act in this way especially when they are applied to coat for example a inflamed intestine or any other inflamed organ.(Slippery Elm).

Herbs - Cranesbill, Chamomile, Eyebright, Feverfew, Ginger, Golden Rod, Ladys Mantle, Licorice, Marshmallow, Meadowsweet, Marigold, Pau D' Arco, Witch Hazel, Wormwood.

Anti-microbial - Helps the body destroy or resist pathogenic micro-organisms.

Herbs - Aniseed, Cayenne, Echinacea, Garlic, Gentian, Marigold, Myrrh, Peppermint, Rosemary, Rue, Sage, Thyme, Wormwood.

Antispasmodic - Prevents or eases spasms and cramps especially of the intestines.

Herbs - Aniseed, Angelica, Chamomile, Fennel, Rosemary, Rue, Sage, Skullcap, St johns Wort, Thyme, Valerian, Vervain.

Anti-viral - Astragalus, Cats claw, Echinacea, Garlic, Myrrh?, Shitake, St Johns Wort, Pau D'Arco.

Anthelmintic - Destroys or expels worms from the digestive system.

Herbs - Garlic, Tansy, Wormwood, Thyme, Rue.

Aperient - Mild laxative.

Herbs - Burdock, Dandelion.

Astringent - Contracts tissue which in turn reduces discharges, these herbs contain tannins. In the digestive system they can be used to stop diarrhea and in the treatment of ulcers. Most astringents also have a anti-bacterial action.

Herbs - Agrimony, Bear Berry, Cranesbill, Comfrey, Eyebright, Golden Rod, Hops, Ladys Mantle, Marigold, Marshmallow, Meadowsweet, Nettles, Raspberry, Sage, Rosemary, Slippery Elm, Shepherds Purse, St Johns Wort, Slippery Elm, Thyme, Witch Hazel, Yarrow.

Bitter - Herbs that taste bitter act as stimulating tonics for the digestive system.

Herbs -Burdock, Feverfew, Gentian, Hops, Horehound, Rue, Tansy, Wormwood.

Carminative - Stimulates peristalsis of the digestive system and relaxes the stomach and helps remove gas and wind from the system. These herbs are usually rich in volatile oils.

Herbs - Aniseed, Angelica, Cayenne, Chamomile, Fennel, Garlic, Ginger, Golden Rod, Hyssop, Horseradish, Juniper, Parsley, Peppermint, Penny Royal, Sage, Rosemary, Tansy, Thyme, Valerian, Wormwood.

Cholagogue - Stimulates the release of bile from the gallbladder which can relieve gallbladder problems, bile is also the body's natural laxative so cholagogues have a laxative effect as well.

Herbs - Agrimony, Blue Flag, Dandelion, Fumitory, Gentian, Marigold, Milk Thistle, Yellow Dock.

Demulcent - Soothes and protects irritated or inflamed internal tissues.

Herbs - Bear Berry, Corn Silk, Coltsfoot, Comfrey, Fenugreek, Licorice, Marshmallow, Milk Thistle, Mullein, Oats, Plantain, Slippery Elm.

Diaphoretic - Aids the skin in the elimination of toxins and produces sweat thus reducing the temperature of fevers.

Herbs - Angelica, Black Cohosh, Cayenne, Chamomile, Elder, Elecampane, Fennel, Garlic, Ginger, Golden Rod, Guaiacum, Hyssop, Lime Blossom, Peppermint, Sarsaparilla, Thyme, Vervain, Yarrow.

Hepatic - Tones and strengthens the liver, may increase the flow of bile.

Herbs - Agrimony, Blue Flag, Dandelion, Fennel, Fumitory, Gentian, Horseradish, Hyssop, Motherwort, Milk Thistle, Vervain, Wormwood, Yarrow.

Laxative - Promotes the evacuation of the bowels.

Herbs - Burdock, Dandelion., Fumitory, Horseradish, Licorice,

Parasiticide - Kills parasites and insects.

Herbs - Aniseed, Rosemary,

Sialagogue - Stimulates the secretion of saliva.

Herbs - Blue flag, Cayenne, Gentian, Ginger.

Respiratory System

Sinusitis

Acute inflammation of the sinuses is relatively uncommon in Goats but a chronic form frequently follows dehorning.

Signs and Symptoms

Shortly after dehorning under unsuitable conditions a suppurative inflammation may set in and progress to a longer lasting purulent sinusitis. There may be head shaking and a rise in temperature in the initial stage, purulent discharge from the nose is seen early on but latter this may be absent. Long standing chronic cases can lead to necrosis of the bone.

Herbal Treatment

Fasting and internal cleansing (see common colds) along with heavy dosing with garlic. Adding ginger to the garlic may help by targeting the garlic to the sinuses and thinning the mucous. Rinsing out the nostrils with1 teaspoon of fresh lemon juice to a cup of tepid water.

Homoeopathic Treatment

Hepar Sulph 6X - Used in low potency the remedy will hasten elimination of purulent material, the pus is usually thin and free flowing. Dose 3 times daily for 4 days.

Hydrastis 30C - Pus bland flowing freely from nostrils. When the discharge is more catarrhal with less purulent involvement. Dose 3 times daily for 6 days

Kali Bich 200C - Long standing cases showing tough stringy yellow discharge. Dose night and morning for 5 days

Silica 200C - Chronic cases showing thin whitish pus associated with affections of the maxillary and nasal bones. Dose night and morning for 5 days.

Arsenic Alb 1M - Discharge acrid tending to excoriate the nostrils, restless, worse after midnight. Dose once daily for 5 days.

Mercurius Corrosivus 200C - Indicated when suspected caries of the bone has taken place, the overlying facial bones being puffy and soft. Pus discharge is greenish and may be tinged with blood. Dose daily for 7 days.

Coryza - Common Cold

Inflammation of the nasal mucous membranes may arise from exposure to cold and damp and frequently attacks Goats that are in poor condition. Coryza has a tendency to extend to the laryngeal and lower respiratory area leading to a possible bronchitis or pneumonia. If there is a lot of respiratory problems in the herd there could be a mineral deficiency of Calcium or Magnesium or they could be out of balance.

Signs and Symptoms

Redness of the mucous membranes of the nose and redness and watering of the eyes are symptoms of nasal catarrh along with a watery discharge that latter can become mucopurulent. In mild cases there is little or no fever but in severe ones it may get high especially in Kids. The animal becomes dull and is not inclined to move about and the appetite may be lost. Swelling of the sub-maxillary lymph glands is frequently seen.

Herbal Treatment

Fast for one or two days, this should then be followed by a cleansing diet which should include abundant carrots (Vitamin A for the lungs), also add a teaspoonful of Paprika to the food. Avoid for some weeks all the nitrogenous foods such as peas and beans and also avoid oats. Dusty hay must be rigidly excluded from the diet; all hay given during the treatment should be well dampened with a solution of water and molasses. Dose with Garlic night and morning and if the throat seems to be sore then give twice daily a drench of honey and elder blossom with sage brew. Honey and lemon juice (Vitamin C) is also excellent for this condition, press the juice of 1 large ripe lemon into half a pint of warm water and stir in 1 tablespoon of honey. The discharging nostrils should be cleansed with a brew of Elder Blossom and Meadowsweet on cotton wool, diluted lemon juice can also be used. The only addition that I would personally make is to add Echinacea to the twice daily garlic dose. Good nursing here could save you from dealing with a far worse condition latter.

Homoeopathic Treatment

Aconitum 6C - Early stages when mucous membrane of the nose is hot and dry, animal thirsty and feverish.

Dose hourly for 4 doses.

Arsenicum Alb 1M - Discharge is acrid, swollen eyelids, thirst for small quantities, restless, worse after midnight, Dose every 2 hours for 4 doses.

Allium Cepa 6C - Discharge bland and watery, eyes red and watery and showing photophobia, dose hourly for 4 doses.

Hepar Sulph 200C - Sneezing with ulceration of the nostrils, discharge thick and purulent, foul smelling, sensitive to pain, resents cold wind. Dose 3 time daily for 2 days.

Nat Mur 1M - Discharge whitish, albuminous looking, there may be violent sneezing, Dose every 2 hours for 4 doses.

Pulsatilla 30C - Loose cough, discharge of greenish foetid matter from nose, sneezing, often worse in morning, affectionate personality. Dose 3 times daily for 3 days.

Dulcamara 200C - When the condition arises as a result of exposure to a fall in temperature after a warm day as frequently happens in late summer or early autumn. Dose every 3 hours for 4 doses.

Cough

While coughing is frequently associated with various pulmonary infections it may arise as a seemingly independent syndrome and takes various forms.

1/. Pleuritic cough - Short and dry and the animal shows pain while coughing.

2/. Bronchitic cough - Starts dry and frequent,

becomes moist and soft.

3/. Simple catarrhal cough - Usually moist and infrequent.

4/. Pneumonic Cough - Frequent, may contain rust colored fibrinous deposits in the sputum.

5/. Stomach or intestinal cough - Various forms dependent on alimentary disorders.

Persistent coughing with no sign of fever can mean lungworm. Any goat that has had lungworm is often left with scared lungs and will cough intermittently for the rest of its life. A course of 500 units of Vitamin E daily for one or 2 weeks could help clear it up as this vitamin minimizes scaring.

Herbal Treatment

Cough is often present in wormy animals long confined in the dusty and vitality impairing atmosphere of stables. I have decided to write the treatment section exactly as it was done in the past and in brackets give you the tinctures used today. For the local relief of the cough give a 1 cup drench of brewed cherry twigs (Wild Cherry Bark Tincture), with one tea spoon of honey and one tea spoon of black treacle added. An alternative and proved excellent drench is a brew of equal parts Pine Needles and Elder twigs, blossoms or leaves (Elder Tincture), 2 handfuls of each of the herbs brewed in a quart of water. Give a drench of one cup. Coltsfoot can replace the Pine or Elder. When mouths are sore or inflamed bath with a brew of Sage. The following Farrier recipe makes a excellent cough drop which could be used for Goats to - Anise seeds one pound (crush seeds to release the oils) , ground ginger one pound, ground licorice one pound and one handful of caraway seeds. Add sufficient treacle to form a mass and roll into balls. Give slightly less than a half ounce of this mixture every morning and fast the Goat for about a hour allowing it time to work.

For Kids

This is a formula that was used in the past for lambs and should be good for using for Kids. What I like about this formula is that it is working in 2 directions at once with one action on worming and the other action on the cough. The formula is equal parts of Garlic, Thyme and Sage made into a strong tea with honey added to make it more palatable, dose morning and evening.

Homoeopathic Treatment

Bryonia 6C - Pleuritic cough, dry, symptoms worse on movement, better from pressure or pressure over the affected area. Dose 3 times daily for 3 days.

Belladonna 30C - Cough accompanied by full pulse, dry cough, hot smooth skin, dilated pupils, nervous symptoms. Dose every 2 hours for 4 doses.

Drosera 6C - Spasmodic coughs of a chronic nature, sometimes associated with asthmatic symptoms worse at night when the animal lies down. Dose every 2 hours for 4 doses.

Nux Vom 6C - Origin in digestive upsets, dry cough, hoarse, spasmodic worse in the morning. Dose 3 times daily for 3 days.

Causticum 30C - Cough relieved by drinking, expectorations scanty. Dose night and morning for 4 days.

Arsenic Alb 1M - Cough worse after midnight, animal restless, thirsty with dry skin, cough worse after drinking even small quantities. Dose night and morning for 4 days.

Spongia 30C - Cough worse on inspiration and worse towards midnight, relieved by drinking, sometimes associated with heart disease. Dose night and morning for 3 days.

Sticta 6C - Cough originates more in trachea, is worse in the evening and during the night and on inspiration. Dose 3 times daily for 3 days.

Bronchitis

Inflammation of the bronchial mucous membranes may arise independently of other illnesses or may be a sequel to another problem or catarrhal state. It may arise simply by exposure to cold dry winds or to damp and cold or may be due to some foreign body irritating the mucous membranes usually as a result of dusty and powdery feeds. Try to remove all causes.

Signs and Symptoms

Loss of appetite, elevation of temperature, pulse becomes full and quick accompanied by a frequent pain full cough but is paroxysmal and incomplete. The inspiration is incomplete short and painful and the expiration is prolonged. Mucous secretion soon becomes purulent and may run from the nose as well as appear in the cough. Rattling respiratory sounds can be herd over the rib area.

Herbal Treatment

The treatment is fairly much the same as Colds and Coughs. Here are a list of some other Herbs that are very good for the treatment of bronchitis - Elecampane (anti-bacterial action as well), Coltsfoot, Grindelia, Mullein, Pleurisy Root, White Horehound and Comfrey. Another thing we can do is to make a steam bag by half filling a sack with bran or sawdust (pine sawdust is the best) then we make a hole in one side of the sack half way down so that hot water can be poured on to the bran or sawdust and to allow a little air to mix with the steam. One tablespoon of Eucalyptus oil can be poured on to the bran-sawdust. Thoroughly soak the contents of the bag with boiling water so a fierce steam is caused to rise. Apply the bag 3 times daily and be careful not to burn the Goat or yourself.

Homoeopathic Treatment

Aconite 6C - Early stages, with hot dry skin, feverish symptoms and anxious expression. Dose hourly for 4 doses

Belladonna 1M - Pulse full and bounding, with dilated pupils, sweating and excitement. Dose every 2 hours for 4 doses.

Ant Tart 30C - Moist cough with threatened pulmonary edema, Rattling sounds may be herd in the chest, respirations increased. Dose 3 times daily for 3 days.

Bryonia 6C - Cough hard and dry, pleura becomes effected, relief from pressure over the ribs. Dose 3 time daily for 3 days.

Dulcamara 6C - Condition has origins from damp surroundings and coughing worse after exertion. Dose 3 times daily for 3 days.

Kali Bich 200C - Phlegm in bronchial tubes difficult to expel, nasal discharge. Dose 3 times daily for 3 days.

Drosera 6C - Coughing becomes spasmodic in character, paroxysms follow one another rapidly. Dose 3 times daily for 4 days.

Spongia 6C - Bouts of coughing eased by eating or drinking, worse by exposure to cold air. Dose 3 times daily for 4 days.

Pneumonia

Inflammation of the lung tissue may appear as a result of exposure to cold and damp and also as a sequel to disease such as Bronchitis. Farm deficiencies of Calcium and Magnesium or these minerals out of balance can cause respiratory problems. Another cause can be over rich unnatural diets given to force up the milk yield which in turn clog the blood stream and cause excessive formation of mucous, the lungs having so much traffic with the blood stream are made unhealthy thereby. The Pus forming bacteria Pneumococci would not be present in large numbers unless there were sufficient mucous and toxic accumulations to nourish them that is why healthy animals don't usually get this problem.

Signs and Symptoms.

A rise in temperature along with a full and hard pulse accompanies coughing, depression and lack of appetite. Can be very cold extremities despite the presence of high fever. The nose may be hot and dry. Respirations are greatly increased and are quick and shallow. The lungs can be panting incessantly and also showing much straining, the ribs are very arched and the eyes much congested. Clear mucous appears on the nostrils which soon give way to a more purulent discharge. Grunting and mouth breathing are present in severe cases. The coat is staring and the skin dry and harsh. The urine is usually diminished in quantity and highly colored and the bowel may be constipated. The animal may stand with the forelegs wide apart to facilitate respiration. In the second stage the temperature drops a bit and the breathing may get a little worse and the cough is frequent and painful. The animal still stands with the forelegs wide apart and elbows turned outwards. If the animal lies down it will try to lie on the sternum. All secretions are more or less suspended and the animal has a haggard appearance and the pulse becomes small and wiry. The extremities are hot and cold alternately. On percussion dullness over the diseased lung is herd indicating consolidation; the lung has now assumed a liver like appearance.

In the third stage if the disease is to terminate favorably the cough becomes loose and the animal improves, the appetite returns and the symptoms rapidly subside. In fatal cases the breath has a peculiar, fetid, cadaverous odor and is taken in short gasps, the horns ears and extremities become cold and clammy and the pulse becomes imperceptible.

Herbal Treatment

Segregate the sick animal from the healthy ones straight away then fast the animal for 2 days to assist the body in cleansing especially the lungs and during this time only give honey and water with powdered Vitamin C added, also you should give the Goat a strong dose of Garlic as this is of tremendous importance in the treatment of respiratory ailments as Garlic exits the body via the mucous membranes especially those of the lungs so its anti-bacterial action will travel there with it. The Garlic dose should be four cloves shredded and brewed in a cup of water with a cup drench being given 3 times a day. Follow the 2 days fasting with a fluid diet of milk, molasses, honey and Slippery Elm powder, 2 tablespoons of each stirred into 1 quart of warm milk. No solid foods should be given while the fever is present. If the fever continues a strong brew of the herb Yarrow can be given so as to promote sweating.

If the lungs are congested another thing we can do is to make a steam bag by half filling a sack with bran or sawdust (pine sawdust is the best) then we make a hole in one side of the sack half way down so that hot water can be poured on to the bran or sawdust and to allow a little air to mix with the steam. One tablespoon of Eucalyptus oil can be poured on to the bran-sawdust. Thoroughly soak the contents of the bag with boiling water so a fierce steam is caused to rise. Apply the bag 3 times daily or at frequent intervals until breathing becomes easier and be careful not to burn the Goat and yourself. Another old recipe is 2 teaspoons full of grated camphor, 3 table spoons of molasses and a little barley flower to bind them. Add the ingredients together and roll them into 8 balls. Give 1 ball twice daily.

Keep the Goat well rugged up and littered up to the belly for warmth but allow plenty of fresh air.

Pat Coleby says Pneumonia will respond well to good nursing and massive doses of Vitamin C with smaller amounts of A, D and especially E which helps heal lung damage. Other herbs to think about are Peppermint for the fever, licorice as a expectorant and Echinacea to build up the immune system.

Homoeopathic Treatment

Aconite 6C - Should always be given first. Dose every half hour for 6 doses.

Antimonium Tart 200C - For moist coughing with patchy distribution of lung lesions, frothy saliva. Dose 3 times daily for 3 days.

Belladonna 1M - Pulse full and bounding, with dilated pupils, sweating and excitement. Dose every 2 hours for 4 doses.

Bryonia 6C - Cough hard and dry, worse on movement and pressure over chest relieves, breathing is difficult and a grunting sound can sometimes be herd with each breath, animal disinclined to move, prefers to lie down. Dose 3 times daily for 2 days.

Drosera 9C - Spasmodic cough is present, gives good results in young Kids.

Phosphorus 200C - A main remedy once hepatisation has set in, pressure resented particularly on the left side, sputum is rust colored, trembling of the body.

Iodum 30C - Hepatisation spreads rapidly, full pulse, absence of pain over chest, temperature remains high, sputum blood streaked. Dose every hour for 4 doses.

Sulphur 30C - Expectoration becomes greenish and purulent, pulse rate decreases towards evening and rises again later in the evening. Dose 3 times daily for 3 days.

Pleurisy

Pleurisy is a inflammation of the serous membrane lining the chest cavity and enveloping the lungs. Injuries to the chest may lead to pleurisy and it may also arise from exposure to cold and damp though is seldom seen as a sole condition in Goats. Acute Pleurisy is usually secondary to Pneumonia or Pericarditis while the chronic form may be associated with lung conditions such as abscess or liver infection.

Signs and Symptoms

The acute form is of sudden onset accompanied by lack of appetite, a rise in temperature and evidence of Pneumonia over the chest wall. In the first stage there is great pain aggravated by movement and the animal may be stiff and still, the pulse is quick and hard with the breathing abdominal and the chest being fixed as far as possible with the inspiration short and jerky and the expiration longer. The pain is caused by the friction of the dry inflamed pleural surfaces of the lung and chest rubbing against each other. At this stage the ear detects a dry friction murmur resembling somewhat the sound made by rubbing to pieces of sole leather together. Pressure between the ribs gives pain and usually causes the animal to grunt. The muzzle is hot and dry. Respirations are increased when secondary to Pneumonia. From here the disease will either get better or worse and in unfavorable cases death occurs during the second or third week from asphyxia or heart failure.

Herbal Treatment

Start the treatment the same as Pneumonia and refer to the other respiratory conditions for treatment for the different symptoms. Below is a summary of how a herbalist would approach the condition using herbal tinctures. If you can get hold of the herbs mentioned below you could make a very effective formula for helping this condition. Read up on each mentioned herb.

Pleurisy is a infection so we shall attack the infection directly with Echinacea and Garlic, fever can also be a large part of pleurisy so we well attack this symptom with the herbs that are called diaphoretics which are herbs used for fevers, some of them are Yarrow, Peppermint and Ginger. As there is a lot of pain with this condition we shall add some demulcent (soothing Herbs) herbs which will hopefully sooth the effected membranes and reduce the pain, a good one here to use is Mullein and I would also be inclined to add Elecampane and Comfrey for its all-round effect. For the Anti-Inflammatory herbs it would be a toss up between Angelica and Golden Rod as these are both good all round herbs and their actions cover most of the symptoms of this disease. So a possible good formula we could make would be Echinacea, Garlic, Mullein, Yarrow and Angelica at about 20% each so it is easy to make up. Try to make your formulas no more than five herbs at a time and try to base them on the actions you need.

Homoeopathic Treatment

Aconite 6C - The early febrile stage. Dose hourly for 4 doses.

Arsenicum 30C - Chronic pleurisy may be relieved by this remedy, useful for cases that are slow to respond. Dose 2 times daily for 7 days.

Belladonna 1M - Pulse full and bounding, with dilated pupils, sweating and excitement. Dose every 2 hours for 4 doses.

Bryonia 30C - Better at rest, pressure over pleural area relieves, cough usually hard and dry, resents movement prefers to lie down, Dose every 2 hours for 4 doses.

Apis 30C - Oedema occurs in pleural cavities, there may be accompanying brisket oedema, urine scanty and high colored. Dose 3 times daily for 3 days

Cantharis 200C - Pleural effusion, mucous expectorated with cough is usually blood stained, severe straining when trying to pass urine.

Kali Carb 200C - Symptoms of pain worse on right side, cough worse in early morning and there is usually a dry throat. Dose 3 times daily for 3 days.

Phosphorus 200C - A main remedy once hepatisation has set in, pressure resented particularly on the left side, sputum is rust colored, trembling of the body, follows well after Aconite or Bryonia.

Sulphur 6C - Use in the convalescent stage of pleurisy. Dose once daily for 6 days.

Herbal Overview Of The Respiratory System

Below are the Actions to think of when dealing with the Respiratory System. As usual isolate the animal and observe. Consider also if the condition is effecting another system. Is there diarrhea, is there any unusual behavior, is there fever, what is the temperature, is the animal anxious etc. Some of the best herbs for this system are Angelica, Coltsfoot, Comfrey, Elder, Elecampane, Eyebright, Fenugreek, Golden Rod, Hyssop, Horehound, Horse Radish, Licorice, Mullein, Myrrh, Plantain, Sage and Thyme.

Anti-biotic - Chaparral, Echinacea, Elecampane, Garlic, Myrrh.

Anti-catarrhal - Helps the body to remove excess catarrhal build ups.

Herbs - Cayenne, Coltsfoot, Cranesbill, Echinacea, Elder, Eyebright, Garlic, Golden Rod, Hyssop, Marshmallow, Mullein, Myrrh, Peppermint, Sage, Thyme, Yarrow.

Anti-inflammatory - Helps the body to combat inflammations. Herbs mentioned under demulcents will often act in this way especially when they coat sore throats and pipe lines.

Herbs - Angelica, Comfrey, Cranesbill, Eyebright, Feverfew, Ginger, Golden Rod, Ladys Mantle, Licorice, Marshmallow.

Anti-microbial - Helps the body destroy or resist pathogenic micro-organisms.

Herbs - Aniseed, Echinacea, Garlic, Myrrh, Peppermint, Plantain, Rosemary, Sage, Thyme.

Antispasmodic - Prevents or eases spasms and cramps.

Herbs - Aniseed, Angelica, Coltsfoot, Fennel, Horehound, Hyssop, Mullein, Rosemary, Sage, Skullcap, Thyme

Anti-viral - Astragalus, Echinacea, Garlic, Myrrh?, Shitake, St Johns Wort, Pau D'Arco.

Anthelmintic - Destroys or expels worms from the digestive system.

Herbs - Garlic, Tansy, Wormwood, Thyme, Rue.

Astringent - Contracts tissue which in turn reduces discharges, these herbs contain tannins.

Herbs - Agrimony, Angelica, Comfrey, Elecampane, Eyebright, Golden Rod, Marshmallow, Mullein,

Myrrh, Plantain, Sage, Rosemary, Shepherds Purse, Thyme.

Demulcent - Soothes and protects irritated or inflamed internal tissues.

Herbs - Coltsfoot, Comfrey, Fenugreek, Licorice, Marshmallow, Mullein, Oats, Plantain.

Diaphoretic - Aids the skin in the elimination of toxins and produces sweat thus reducing the temperature of fevers.

Herbs - Angelica, Cayenne, Elder, Elecampane, Fennel, Garlic, Ginger, Golden Rod, Hyssop, Peppermint, Thyme, Yarrow.

Expectorant - Supports the body in the removal of excess mucous from the respiratory system and helps in the control of coughs.

Herbs -Angelica, Aniseed, Coltsfoot, Comfrey, Elder, Elecampane, Fennel, Fenugreek, Garlic, Hyssop, Horehound, Licorice, Marshmallow, Mullein, Myrrh, Plantain, Sweet Violets, Thyme.

Febrifuge - Helps the body to bring down fevers.

Herbs - Cayenne, Elder Flowers, Hyssop, Marigold, Penny Royal, Peppermint, Plantain, Raspberry, Sage, Thyme, Vervain.

Immune Booster - Astragalus, Echinacea, Reshi, Shitake.

Pectoral - Has a general strengthening and healing effect on the respiratory system.

Herbs - Aniseed, Coltsfoot, Comfrey, Elder, Garlic, Hyssop, Licorice, Mullein, Horehound.

The Nervous System

Encephalitis

This term implies inflammation of the brain or any inflammatory lesion occurring to the brain tissue. It leads to loss of nervous function. Most cases are related to bacterial or viral infection though injury can be a cause.

Signs and Symptoms

Encephalitis is usually accompanied by fever, toxemia, anorexia, depression and tachycardia. Normal stimuli can produce exaggerated responses, the animal being easily startled. There may be convulsions accompanied by squinting of eyes and clamping of jaws. Excitement may be a early sign, brain involvement is evident by bellowing, head shaking and staring pupils and maybe head pressing.

Herbal Treatment

Herbal treatment could be too slow for a fast acting disease as this but consider Garlic ,Echinacea and Myrrh for bacterial and viral infections. Another herb to look at is St Johns Wort because it is a Nervine anti-viral. Essential oils can cross the blood brain barrier and could be a fast way of getting into the area so try maybe Garlic oil ,Lavender oil, Myrrh, Thyme or Eucalyptus diluted and rubbed in the head area as these are all anti microbials. I have not heard of essential oils being used for this condition but as a last desperate resort I would try it. Homoeopathy is the better action to take as it is faster acting then herbal medicine and I would also give Vitamin C injections straight away a 50cc intramuscularly with half the dose on each side of the body. Most vets would give you not much hope.

Homoeopathic Treatment

Aconite 6C - If seen early enough this should be given in the febrile stage. Dose hourly for 4 hours.

Arnica 30C - Give this remedy if the cause of the condition was from injury.

Belladonna 1M - This remedy is useful for deranged nerve conditions, there is a accompanying full bounding pulse, fever, dilated pupils and a smooth hot skin, convulsions, excitement and head pressing. Dose hourly for 4 doses.

Stramonium 30C - Indicated when signs of vertigo appear, such as a tendency to stagger and fall sideways, the eyes are usually wide open and staring. Dose 4 times daily for 2 days.

Hyoscyamus 200C - Indications for this remedy include frequent head shaking and a tendency to muscular twitching. There may be signs of abdominal discomfort. Dose 3 times daily for 3 days.

Phosphorus 200C - Useful in less acute cases showing a tendency to reoccur. The animal becomes unsteady after rising. Dose night and morning for one week.

Zincum Met 6C - Indicated where there is a tendency for the head to roll from side to side. Hyperaesthesia and hyperexcitability are present, easily startled, paddling of feet may occur. Dose 3 times daily for 3 days.

Meningitis

Inflammation of the meninges is usually secondary to viral or bacterial infection. Infection may enter through a penetrating wound but more often the infection is spread through the blood, Kids can become infected from the umbilical cord.

Signs and Symptoms

This condition is characterized by fever and muscle rigidity. Restlessness and head shaking are common which can go on to pressing the head against any suitable object. Sensitivity of the skin is a common symptom, there is a retraction of the head and stiffness of the neck muscles, paresis of the hindquarters is common. There can be increased nervous activity and so increased response to pain, excitement or depression and a raised body temperature.

Herbal Treatment

This is the same as Encephalitis. Meningitis is a fast acting acute infection and herbal remedies may act to slow to control the condition but would be very helpful in assisting the recovery.

The best action here is to call the vet and hope that he has the right antibiotics to target the cause.

Refer to Encephalitis and use the treatment given there.

Homoeopathic Treatment

Aconite 6C - Should be given in the early febrile stage, the animal usually looks anxious and there is a rapid short pulse. Dose hourly for 4 hours.

Apis 6C - The acute form is sometimes associated with edema of the meninges and this remedy will benefit such cases. Dose every half hour for 5 doses.

Belladonna 1M - The indications for this remedy are a accompanying encephalitis with dilated pupils and a throbbing pulse, the skin is smooth and hot, sweating is common. Dose 2 hourly.

Zincum Met 6C - Indicated where there is a tendency for the head to roll from side to side. Hyperaesthesia and hyperexcitability are present, easily startled, paddling of feet may occur. Dose 3 times daily for 3 days.

Bryonia 6C - Indicated in cases showing vertigo, the animal resents movement and there is excessive dryness of the mucous membranes eg seen in the mouth where the lips show a parched appearance and there is great thirst. Dose 3 times daily for 3 days.

Veratum 30C - The legs and ears are icy cold, there is convulsive trembling of the whole body or there is a reeling, staggering motion, and the animal plunges violently and falls down head foremost.

Cuprum Met 30C - A useful remedy when convulsions are associated more with meningitis then with encephalitis. The head usually assumes a lowered posture and there may be attempts to press it against any suitable object.

Cerebral Oedema

This condition sometimes accompanies brain diseases

of ruminants or may be a result of injury.

Signs and Symptoms

Blindness is a early symptom followed by convulsions and muscle tremors along with stretching of the neck and back. Muscle in-coordination soon sets in and the animal may become recumbent with increased convulsions.

Homoeopathic Treatment

Apis 6C - The acute form is sometimes associated with edema of the meninges and this remedy will benefit such cases. Dose every half hour for 5 doses.

Arnica 30C - Give this remedy if the cause of the condition was from injury.

Belladonna 1M - This remedy is useful for deranged nerve conditions, there is a accompanying full bounding pulse, fever, dilated pupils and a smooth hot skin, convulsions, excitement and head pressing. Dose hourly for 4 doses.

Strychninum 200C - Indicated when stretching of neck and back is prominent. Dose daily for 7 days.

Herbal Overview Of The Nervous System

One of the most important herbs in this system is Hypericum also known as St Johns Wort. This herb is anti-viral, probably antibacterial, anti-inflammatory, a sedative and one of our main first aid remedies for wounds which helps relieve pain and can kill the tetanus bacteria and this is only mentioning a part of its uses, always consider this when there are problems with this system especially if you don't know what the problem is. Another good herb for rebuilding this system is Oats which is a Nervine tonic also think of Valerian which is our main Tranquillizer but also a good tonic for this system. A lot of the herbs mentioned below are used in a lot of other systems as well so when you want the action of a Nervine to use in another system try to match the herb to one used in that system as well.

Antispasmodic - Prevents or eases spasms and cramps.

Herbs - Aniseed, Angelica, Black Cohosh, Chamomile, Fennel, Horehound, Hyssop, Lime Blossom, Mistletoe, Motherwort, Rosemary, Rue, Sage, Skullcap, St johns Wort, Thyme, Valerian, Vervain.

Nervine - Has a beneficial effect on the nervous system, acts like a tonic to this system.

Herbs - Black Cohosh, Chamomile, Hops, Lime Blossoms, Mistletoe, Motherwort, Oats, Peppermint, Rosemary, Skullcap, St Johns Wort, Tansy, Thyme, Valerian, Vervain, Wormwood.

Sedative - Calms the nervous system and reduces stress and nervousness throughout the body.

Herbs - Black Cohosh, Chamomile, Hops, Hyssop, Motherwort, Skullcap, St Johns Wort, Valerian , Vervain.

The Urinary System

Acute Nephritis   (Inflammation of the Kidney)

This condition is rarely by itself in Goats there is usually a cause such as Septicaemic infections which are brought to the kidney by the blood. The condition may also arise as a sequel to mastitis, metritis or some other septic condition. Chemical poisoning frequently leads to Nephritis.

Signs and Symptoms

There is a initial rise in temperature with accelerated pulse followed by anorexia and possibly increased respiration. Tenderness over the kidney area is common, the urine itself may contain blood, pus, mucous and proteins may be present, dry hot muzzle, burning at the roots of the horns and ears and suspended rumination.

The Goat may stand with back arched and the hind legs extended backwards and outwards and there may be frequent urination of small amounts of highly colored urine with maybe occasional difficulty in passing. When made to move the patient does so with hesitation and groaning especially if turned in a narrow circle.

Herbal Treatment

The first thing to do here is to try and establish the cause and remove that. Parsley, Chicory and Horsetail are the main herbs to use here. Four handfuls of herb boiled and brewed in one quart of water with 2 tablespoons of honey added when the brew has cooled to tepid. Give a cupful as a drench maybe 3 times a day.

Other herbs to consider for kidney problems are Bearberry, Buchu and Corn silk. If you think the condition may have been caused by infection think of Echinacea and Garlic. Remember this is a life threatening problem and a vet should be called because there may have to be some very quick decisions made.

The convalescent diet should include pulped carrots. Barley is the best cereal to be used for kidney cases, feed also couch grass.

Homoeopathic Treatment

Apis 6C - Renal edema in the acute form, urine shows albuminous casts. Dose every 2 hours for 4 doses.

Arsenicum 1M - Scanty urine showing albumen content and drops of blood, the animal is restless and thirsty for small amounts, there is a harsh dry coat, symptoms are worse after midnight. Dose every 3 hours for 4 doses.

Belladonna 1M - Acute cases showing excitement and dilated pupils, full bounding pulse and hot smooth skin, straining to pass urine which is scanty and loaded with phosphates, blood in urine is common. Dose every 2 hours for 4 doses.

Beberis 6C - Tenderness over the kidneys and sacral region accompanies frequent urination, the urine is cloudy and contains a reddish sediment. Dose 3 hourly for 4 doses.

Mercurius Sol 30C - Urine scanty with greenish mucous sediment which may contain pus and blood. Urine is dark colored. Dose 3 times daily for 4 days.

Lycopodium 200C - Urine profuse during the night, tendency to retention with thick reddish sediment. Dose night and morning for 5 days.

Phosphorus 200C - Acute cases showing blood in urine, blood is diffused throughout the urine giving a brownish appearance. Dose night and morning for 3 days.

Nat Mur 200C - Chronic cases showing a pale urine of low specific gravity, there is usually salt retention leading to thirst and anemia. Dose night and morning for one week.

Urolithiasis - (Stones and Gravel)

This condition may arise from to heavily mineralized boar water and stasis of the urine. Various factors contribute including dry feeding and lack of water. A study of the makeup of a passed stone may give you a clue as to the cause of the problem.

Signs and Symptoms

Obvious difficulty in passing urine which is scanty and blood stained. Signs of pain include kicking at belly and looking around at flanks. Severe attacks are called renal colic and this may be shown by frequent uneasy shifting of the hind limbs, shaking or twisting of the tail, looking around at the flanks and lying down and rising again at short intervals without apparent cause. In bad cases inflammation of the kidneys may set in. There can be lots of complications with stones with some of the worst being blocked ureters which are between the kidney and bladder and then there may be a blockage after the bladder as is common in male Goats

Herbal Treatment

The same treatment as for kidney disorders should be followed but first try and establish the cause. Couch grass should always be added to the Parsley or any of the other herbs given for the cure of Nephritis. Warm milk and molasses is highly beneficial for this complaint fortified with Slippery Elm Bark (one heaped tablespoon full to the quart). Also look at the herbs Cleavers, Bearberry, Gravel Root and Chaparral which are all anti lithics. Horsetail is another good herb for stones as it is high in silica and this may help to break up the stone. It is also wise to add some demulcents to sooth the pain caused by gravel scraping its way down, some good ones for this system are Corn silk and Marshmallow. Pat Coleby says if the problem is from highly mineralized water add a little apple cider vinegar in the food and stones do not occur. The amount needed is surprisingly small, just a desert spoon every few days would be enough.. Two teaspoons full can also be given daily for two or three days as it may help dissolve the stones and flush the bits out. Prevention is better than cure.

Homoeopathic Treatment - See also cystitis

Lycopodium 200C - Hepatic symptoms with blood

stained urine containing red sediment, the early stages of stone formation. Dose night and morning for 7 days.

Sarsaparilla 6C - Pain at the beginning and end of urination especially at the end, Urine contains gravely deposits and is slimy. Dose 3 times daily for 3 days.

Urtica Urens 6X - Thickens the urine and removes the tendency to gravel formation by removing the basic salts that help form it, it will also increase the quantity of urine passed, there may be a skin rash, give one dose 3 times daily for 10 days.

Calc Phos 30C - A good constitutional remedy which will help regulate the calcium and phosphate metabolism and so prevent the formation of phosphates, it should be given as a routine remedy in young animals up till the age of one. One dose weekly for 8 weeks.

Mag Mur 6C - May help in preventing some forms of stones and may be given as a routine remedy if the urine shows suspicious deposits and there are other signs of stone formation.

Cystitis

Inflammation of the bladder can arise from a infection in some other part of the urinary system and a infection here can also travel up the ureters and infect the kidneys if not looked after. Cystitis can also arise as a result of stones and gravel damaging the delicate tissue and leaving it open for infection. This condition can be acute or chronic with the acute condition usually caused by bacteria and the chronic caused by gravel and stones. Another common cause is difficult birthing leading to a infection especially from poor hygiene.

Signs and symptoms

Frequent urination is the commonest sign with the urine often containing blood. There may be considerable difficulty in passing urine. Arching of the back and signs of pain are evident such as kicking at the abdomen and urinating while lying down. There may be constant tail wagging as if on heat and there could be swelling of the vulva.

Herbal Treatment

The main herbs we use in cystitis are the urinary antiseptics with the best ones being Bearberry and Buchu. Cranberry juice is a good urinary antiseptic to. To the antiseptics we add demulcents which sooth the irritated tissues with the best one for this condition being Corn Silk. You could add to the formula Gravel Root and Chaparral if you think the cause of the condition could be from urinary stones or gravel which tend to scratch and inflame the pipelines leaving them open to infection. Other herbs to consider are Angelica, Yarrow, Agrimony, Cleavers, Damiana, Golden Rod, Juniper, Plantain and Shepherds Purse. These herbs can be mixed as tinctures and then have water added to bring them up to a cup size drench or could be mixed together in dry form and then made into a tea.

Homoeopathic Treatment.

Aconite 6C - In the early febrile involvement when pulse and respiration are increased, frequent ineffectual and painful attempts to urinate, pain on pressure of bladder. Dose ever hour for 4 doses.

Cantharis 30C - Much straining and scanty amounts of bloody urine, there is hyperexcitability and signs of sexual irritability, signs of abdominal pain prominent. Dose night and morning in chronic cases for one week, in acute cases give one dose every hour for 4 doses.

Colocynthis 1M - Arching of the back and kicking at the abdomen suggest this remedy. Signs of severe pain are present. Dose every hour for 4 doses.

Nux Vom 30C - When ineffectual urging is associated with digestive upsets. Good to use if Cantharis does not work. Dose 3 times daily for 2 days.

Dulcamara 30C - Catarrhal cystitis resulting from exposure to cold or damp, urine contains a thick mucus or purulent sediment. Dose 3 times daily for 3 days.

Causticum 30C - A useful remedy in the recurrent or chronic form and is especially adapted to the older animal. Follows well after Cantharis which may be needed if acute symptoms flare up in the chronic form.

Uva Ursi 3X - Useful in chronic cystitis, urine is slimy, pain and straining are common. Dose 3 times daily for 7 days.

Herbal Overview Of The Urinary System

Most infections get to the kidneys via the blood for the kidneys are the main filter of the blood removing wastes and water. Other infections can start off as cystitis and travel up the ureter and infect the kidney that way so you must always consider both ways. Always ask yourself is the infection traveling from the kidney down or the bladder up? If you think it is the kidney put a leash on the animal and walk them in tight circles one way and then the other. If the animal complains it is probably the kidney. Urinary antiseptics are good for this system whether for treating infection or preventing it as in cases of stones scraping the sides as they go down leaving a wound ripe for infection. Also think of Cranberry for this system as it coats the pipes and stops bacteria getting a foot hold literally.

Herbal Actions For The Urinary System

Anti-biotic - Chaparral, Echinacea, Garlic, Myrrh, Pau D' Arco.

Anti-inflammatory - Helps the body to combat inflammations.

Herbs - Cats Claw, Chaparral , Cleavers, Cranesbill, Eyebright, Ginger, Golden Rod, Guaiacum, Liquorice, Marshmallow, Pau D' Arco.

Anti-lithic - Prevent the formation of stones or gravel in the urinary system and helps the body to remove them.

Herbs - Bearberry, Corn Silk, Chaparral , Gravel Root, Horsetail.

Anti-microbial - Helps the body destroy or resist pathogenic micro-organisms.

Herbs - Echinacea, Garlic, Juniper, Myrrh,

Astringent - Contracts tissue which in turn reduces discharges, these herbs contain tannins.

Herbs - Agrimony, Cranesbill, Chaparral, Golden Rod, Horsetail, Shepherds Purse.

Cystitis - Agrimony, Bearberry, Buchu, Celery Seed, Corn Silk, Gravel Root, Golden Rod, Horsetail, Plantain,

Demulcent - Soothes and protects irritated or inflamed internal tissues.

Herbs - Bearberry, Corn Silk, Licorice, Marshmallow, Plantain, Slippery Elm.

Diuretic - Increases the secretion and elimination of urine.

Herbs - Agrimony Angelica, Bear Berry, Blue Flag, Burdock, Buchu, Broom, Coltsfoot, Chaparral, Corn Silk, Dandelion Leaves, Elder, Fumitory, Golden Rod, Guaiacum, Gravel Root, Hawthorn, Horseradish, Horsetail, Juniper, Lime Blossom, Nettles, Pau D' Arco, Penny Royal, Plantain, Parsley, Shepherds Purse, Sarsaparilla, Yarrow.

Urinary Antiseptics - These herbs have a antiseptic action as they pass through the system.

Herbs - Angelica, Bearberry, Buchu, Corn Silk,

Golden Rod, Shepherds Purse, Yarrow.

NOTES

The Muscular Skeletal System

Myositis

Inflammation of the muscle tissue may have its origin in a open wound or infection, or it may be the result of severe straining.

Signs and Symptoms

Local heat in the muscle is a early sign, followed by stiffness or lameness if leg muscles are involved. Febrile signs will accompany infectious conditions.

Herbal Treatment

If the cause is from bacterial infection then we would use our immune boosting herbs so as to start fighting the infection, these are Echinacea, Myrrh and Garlic. If inflammation is present treat with anti inflammatories especially the ones that are pain killers - Willow bark and Devils Claw. If the inflammation was caused by injury try some of the First Aid remedies such as a compress of Arnica Lotion. Don't forget to look at the Homoeopathic First Aid remedies.

Homoeopathic Treatment.

Arnica 30C - Should always be given in the early inflammatory stage. Doses every 2 hours for 2 doses.

Apis 6C - Give if edema accompanies inflammation. Dose every 3 hours for 4 doses.

Rhus Tox 6C - Indicated when the animal gains relief from movement even though the initial movement is painful, symptoms may be more on the left side of the body then the right, indicated when severe wetting or prolong dampness is associated with the onset of the symptoms.

Bryonia 30C - Movement is resented when Bryonia is indicated. The animal will seek to lie on the affected muscles because pressure on them gives ease, warmth is usually useful also.

Hepar Sulph 30C - Infection from a open scratch or wound. Dose 3 times daily for 3 days.

Osteoarthritis

Degenerative joint disease of a non-inflammatory origin where the articular cartilages become eroded and bony exostoses that occur at the margin of the joints. All though age plays a part there can be other causes such as systemic or metabolic disturbances. Progressive mild inflammation in the joint over a period of time is more likely to produce osteoarthritis than any other predisposing factor. Osteoarthritis particularly affects the load bearing bones of the body. Being overweight adds to the wear and tear of the joints. Once the cartilage degenerates the cushioning effect is lost within the joint and the joint capsule now becomes involved and the situation becomes worse.

Bucks kept in small yards with little exercise may develop arthritis in the hip joints especially when feed large quantities of Lucerne hay as well as supplements this happens because Lucerne is high in calcium plus the Buck is probably getting calcium supplements. Compare this to the Doe who is losing calcium in milk and the making of kids, so always check the diet when arthritis is present.

Too much calcium as well as to less can cause arthritis.

Signs and Symptoms

Lameness is the main sign and it could involve several joints. Constant running on concrete and inattention to hooves which can become so overgrown and painful that goats will walk on their knees (thus damaging them) can cause arthritis. In older animals with arthritis the joints may ankylose, especially the neck and elbow joints and the animal may walk with a stilted action and the neck may be extended as that of a tortoise. Sometimes you can hear the hip and pelvic joints when the Goat walks.

Herbal Treatment

Nutrition wise for the early stages you can give calcium, Vitamin D, magnesium and manganese so as to try to stop the condition from getting worse this is of course after you have checked to see if the diet and to much calcium was the cause. Glucosamine and Chondroitin Sulphate can help stimulate the rebuilding of cartilage and help in the early stages of arthritis.

Arthritis with lots of pain and inflammation needs the use of the anti-inflammatory herbs, good ones to use for this condition are Meadowsweet, Devils Claw and Willow bark as these act as good pain killers as well. Other herbs to use are the alteratives which clean out the area and the system some good ones are Burdock,

Garlic, Sarsaparilla and Chaparral which has a antioxidant action as well. Diuretic herbs are also used for this condition as they help to remove the metabolic waste and toxins which usually result from the constant inflammation and help the kidneys flush this waste out, some good ones are Celery seed, Juniper (these two are best used together) and Dandelion leaf. Other herbs to look at for arthritis are Black Cohosh, Cats Claw, Guaiacum, Nettles, Wild Yam and Yellow dock. Add Licorice to the formula at about 10% as this will help in the assimilation of the formula into the body.

Homoeopathic Treatment

Not an easy condition to treat. Start treatment as early as possible so as to slow down deterioration. Useful remedies for the early inflammatory stages are.

Rhus Tox 6C - This remedy is indicated when the animal's symptoms are eased after a short period of movement. There may be initial stiffness on first moving.

Bryonia 6C - The indications for this remedy are the opposite of the above, the animal prefers to remain still and any movement causes distress and sometimes acute pain evidenced by the animal crying out.

Calc Flour 30C - May be needed in the latter stages once the exostoses and joint swellings develop. The carpus is the main joint affected when this remedy is indicated. There may be accompanying cystic tumors around the joint.

Rhus Tox 1M - This can be given in the latter stages to help with the symptoms of pain when the animal moves.

Arthritis Due To Infection

This is caused by pyogenic bacteria getting in the joint mainly from injury the main organisms are Streptococci and Staphylococci . Kids can get this infection through their navel cords and it comes on 2 to 3 weeks after birth.

Signs and Symptoms

There may be a initial temperature rise and febrile signs may develop. The affected joint becomes swollen, stiff, tense and hot due to inflammation. Pain is obvious by the onset of severe lameness. Examination may reveal the presence of punctures on the skin and the appearance of a purulent exudate. In Kids there may be suppurating joints of the fetlocks, knees and hocks.

Herbal Treatment

For this condition think of our infection fighting herbs such as Echinacea, Garlic and Myrrh. If the skin is broken and you think the infection got in this way apply a lotion or cream of Calendula and Hypericum to the area. To our infection fighting herbs you can add some of the anti inflammatories, alteratives and diuretics that are mentioned in Osteo-Arthritis. Add Licorice to the formula at about 10% as this will help in the assimilation of the formula into the body.

Homoeopathic Treatment

Aconitum 30C - This should be given as soon as possible in the early febrile stage.

Ferrum Phos 6C - This also is a good remedy for the initial feverish stage more often indicated when throat symptoms accompany the invasive process.

Belladonna 30C - Indicated when the patient presents a excitable picture with dilated pupils, throbbing arteries and a hot skin.

Bryonia 6C - Symptoms worse for movement, relief from pain on pressure over the joint and a possible involvement with the respiratory tract. The joint is usually extremely hard and tense.

Apis Mel 6C - If the synovial sheaf of the joint becomes edematous indicated by swelling this remedy may help. The patient is made worse by heat in any form and does not drink much.

Ledum 6C - The remedy of choice if the arthritis has been caused by the penetration of a sharp object giving rise to a puncture wound.

Iodum 6C - This is a remedy which sometimes gives good results in the less acute case especially when the joint pains are worse at night. The patient is often thin with a voracious appetite and the skin is dry and withered looking.

Rhus Tox 6C - The indications for this remedy are relief from movement although there may be initial stiffness on rising. There may be accompanying skin symptoms of a vesicular itchy nature.

Silica 30C - This remedy is indicated in the more

chronic case. There may be involvement of neighboring lymphatic glands showing cold abscesses.

Caprine Arthritis Encephalitis (Big Knee)

Known simply as CAE this virus disease has only been known for a short time. The virus which causes it is a member of the retrovirus group (associated with diseases such as Feline Leukaemia) and can be transmitted by a infected Doe through the colostrum to her Kid. Young Kids are at risk from older infected animals. The young animals may show paralysis while in adults the disease is characterized by arthritis. It is unusual for Goats once infected to clear themselves of infection, a carrier state being normal. The disease is more common in Dairy Goats. Take care that any new Goats introduced to the herd are not infected.

Signs and Symptoms

Young Kids affected by the encephalitic form show varying symptoms depending on the virulence of the infection eg mild cases may present with little more than staggering or a uncertain gait, while more severe cases rapidly progress to paralysis. Hind limb weakness is often a early sign but soon all legs become involved within a few weeks.

In the adult animal early arthritis develops and becomes progressively worse. A harsh dry coat develops in the early stages when infected Kids grow to maturity. The carpel (knee) joints are the ones most at risk. Underlying tissues such as tendon sheaths and ligaments also become involved. Affected joints remain free of secondary infections. The most common symptoms are swelling of the knees with accompanying lameness with maybe a slow wasting away. This is a Auto Immune type of disease. There is no treatment or vaccine available.

Herbal Treatment

Here all we can really do is try to attack the virus itself with herbs like Echinacea, Myrrh, Garlic, PauD'arco, Vitamin C and maybe even try L -lysine and hope for the best. The arthritis symptoms can be treated as under arthritis. Cats Claw and Devils Claw may be worth looking at but with a disease like this you will just have to experiment. There may be a link between CAE and a lack of copper in the diet.

Homoeopathic Treatment

Conium 30C - Early hind leg weakness will be helped by this remedy. Dose once daily for 10 days.

Gelsemium 30C - The affinity of this plant is the nervous system which produces varying degrees of motor paralysis, there is usually weakness and muscle tremors. Dose 3 times daily

Stramonium 200C - Staggering and falling towards the left side indicates this remedy. Dose 3 times weekly for 4 weeks.

Rhus Tox 6C - If the arthritis state has not progressed to far this remedy may give some relief.

Dose 3 times a day for 21 days

Herbal Overview Of The Muscular Skeletal System

For bruising think about Arnica in a lotion and use the Homoeopathic dose internally, for broken bones think about Comfrey as its old name is knit bone. For arthritis and rheumatism use your Anti Rheumatics, Anti Inflammatorys, and Analgesics but also think of Celery Seed as this is called the acid remover and another herb to think of is Meadowsweet as this herb is called the acid balancer. It is usually the high acid in the system that irritates the joints and starts the inflammation so these 2 herbs could remove the cause for the condition; also consider diet as a diet high in protein will create a lot of acid waste. For blood borne bacterial infections think of the Alteratives (blood cleansers) and Anti Bacterials especially our main ones Garlic and Echinacea. If there is damage to the joints use a nutritional supplement with these 3 together - Glucosamine Sulphate, Chondroitin and MSM as these together will help rebuild the joints.

Herbal Actions For The Muscular Skeletal System

Alterative - Herbs that gradually restore proper function to the body, they increase health and vitality. They were once known as the blood cleansers.

Herbs - Black Cohosh, Blue Flag, Burdock, Chaparral, Echinacea, Garlic, Nettles, Pau D'Arco ,Sarsaparilla, Yellow Dock.

Analgesic - Herbs that reduce pain.

Herbs - Black Cohosh, Chamomile, Hops, Meadowsweet, Pau D'Arco, Peppermint, Skullcap, St Johns Wort, Valerian.

Anti-biotic - Chaparral, Echinacea, Garlic, Myrrh, Pau D' Arco.

Antispasmodic - Prevents or eases spasms and cramps.

Herbs - Angelica, Black Cohosh, Chamomile, Skullcap, St johns Wort, Valerian.

Anti-inflammatory - Helps the body to combat inflammations.

Herbs - Cats Claw, Devils Claw, Chaparral , Feverfew, Ginger, Guaiacum, Licorice, Meadowsweet, Pau D' Arco, Sarsaparilla, St Johns Wort, Willow Bark.

Anti-viral - Astragalus, Cats claw, Echinacea, Garlic, Myrrh?, St Johns Wort, Pau D'Arco.

Anti-Rheumatic - Angelica, Burdock, Black Cohosh, Chaparral, Cats Claw, Celery Seed, Dandelion, Garlic, Guaiacum, Nettles, Willow Bark, Yellow Dock.

Rubefacient - Causes a gentle local irritation to the skin which stimulates the capillaries to open increasing the blood flow.

Herbs - Cayenne, Garlic, Ginger, Horseradish, Nettles, Peppermint Oil, Rosemary Oil, Rue.

The Skin

Foot Rot

There are 2 types of foot rot in Goats. The first is called common often found when the sheep are in damp or marshy types of areas and the other is more virulent and very contagious. Symptoms of both are alike in the beginning but if you find out latter that it is the virulent condition separate the involved animals for at least a month. Foot Rot is a bacterial infection. In some places notification of this disease in compulsory.

Signs and Symptoms - Slight lameness is the early sign with extreme lameness showing a severe condition and in this case you will see the animal grazing while on its knees in good pastures. The main symptoms are severe pain and lameness. It can start with small chapped areas between the spaces of the toes or it may look red and inflamed. The horn and the hoof become soft and crumbly and gives off a unpleasant odor, there may be a gray pasty scum between the claws. In advanced cases the horn of the toes may separate from the feet.

Move animals to dry clean smooth pasture for treatment and recovery.

Prevention - Avoid damp and marshy pastures especially in the change of seasons, remember Goats are hill dwelling animals. Also never put a new animal straight into the herd always quarantine for a while. If animals have to be kept in damp areas inspect feet regularly.

Herbal Treatment - The presence of foot rot indicates that the land is not well. Diet wise Juliette de Bairacli Levy recommends a purge and then build up the animals on with good foods such as oats, wheat, given crushed and mixed with molasses and pulped carrots. Dose animals with garlic. For area treatment wash in a bath of mild detergent with disinfectant and lots of salt added. After area is clean inspect and trim hooves carefully. Bathe with a lotion of calendula and Hypericum. Hypericum (St Johns Wort) in this case should help pain. Apply a cream to the area made up of Calendula and Hypericum. Do this twice each day and give the Homoeopathic remedies indicated. Keep animals in a dry clean sick bay for a few days so you can monitor progress.

Homoeopathic Treatment

Kreosotum - This is one of the main remedies as it has a profound action on diseased horn and surrounding tissues. Give 200C twice weekly for 4 to 6 weeks.

Hepar Sulph - The pain associated with the condition should be relieved by this remedy. Give 1M daily for seven days.

Silicea - Once the acute state has been relieved follow on with this remedy as it will quickly build up hard healthy horn which will more easily resist subsequent reinfection. Give 200C twice weekly for 6 weeks.

Foot Rot Nosode - A 30C potency of the nosode should be given at the beginning of autumn and then again in spring twice weekly for 6 weeks. This should hopefully act as a preventative. In acute conditions give daily with the selected remedy for 7 days.

Scabby Mouth (Orf)

This is a viral disease that affects Goats and Sheep and is highly contagious. Usually encountered in early summer though there is a severe form that can show at other times. Most age groups are affected. Goats can develop a life time immunity after the initial exposure. Thistles that puncture lips and feet can predispose Goats to a severe outbreak.

Caution - This disease can pass on to humans and if it does it is usually seen on the hands and arms and is known as Orf.

Herbal Treatment - Use a Calendula and Hypericum Lotion (1 to 10) on affected area. Be careful not to come into contact as humans can be infected. Mix up lotion and put in a spray bottle and gently spray affected areas.

Symptoms - Raw bleeding areas appear around the muzzle which then quickly turn into large scabby lesions. Thick brown scabs form on the lips, mouth and nasal areas and or on the teats and the skin above the hoof, particularly between and above the heels. When these dry the scabs tend to fall off and healing follows. In Does there could be a reduced milk output. Healing is spontaneous in 3 to 4 weeks unless delayed by fly strike or a secondary infection. Loss of condition accompanies the process due to the animal's reluctance to eat because of the pain in the mouth.

Homoeopathic Treatment

Acid Nit 200C - This is the main remedy to consider in any eczematous condition appearing at the junction of skin and any mucous membrane. This should help the problem and limit the spread. Give 200C daily for 7 days.

Rhus Tox - For the so called malignant form of Orf which arises on the udder and surrounding skin on older Ewes. Give 1M daily for 14 days.

Orf Nosode - Give this along with the other remedies. Give 30C daily for 5 days.

Ringworm

Ringworm lesions in goats are caused by the fungal agents. This condition is a fungal infection that is highly contagious between animals and can be passed on to humans.

Symptoms - Reddish circular lesions appear on the skin especially in the abdominal area and latter progress to a dry scabby lesion. Other common areas are behind the ears and the back of the neck. They first appear as brownish nodules that enlarge and join together to form a large roughened area with dry crusts around the edges. There may be itching in the area.

Herbal Treatment

Ringworm is a fungal infection which usually attacks when the immune system is weakened by stress or exhaustion. Fungi thrive in damp, dark and confined places. If you think the immune system is run down you can give Echinacea, zinc, and vitamin C and you might as well give garlic as this has a anti-fungal action. Externally treatment can be a lotion of calendula 1 to 5 in strength for cleaning the area and around it. Stronger anti fungals may be necessary as this can sometimes be a very stubborn condition to get rid of. Garlic is a stronger anti-fungal and you can use this externally and internally at the same time. Another strong anti-fungal we have is Tea Tree oil which can be put on neat to the infected area. Other herbs that have been traditionally used for this condition are Herb Robert, Lemon juice, Rue and Walnut.

Treatment

Raise immunity.

Calendula lotion 1 to 5 strength on and around the affected area. (can mix with garlic)

Tea tree oil - strong anti-fungal dab on to the affected area neat.

Garlic externally on effected area and latter if problem is not resolving take internally.

Raw lemon juice applied twice daily.

Other herbs to look at are Burdock, Elder, Sarsaparilla, Myrrh and Rue.

Homoeopathic Treatment

Bacillinum 200C - This nosode has a proven record in the treatment of ringworm. 2 doses at two week intervals with sepia 6C.

Sepia 200C - Use with the above remedy in bad out

breaks and by itself in mild outbreaks. Dose once per week for 4 weeks.

Tellurium 30C - Twice a day for one week especially when lesions tend to be equally distributed on either side of the body.

Chrysarobinum 6C - 3 times a day for 5 days, when the disease has progressed to the crusty stage.

Note - Animals that are susceptible to ringworms are usually deficient in copper. Give a Kelp Supplement.

Goat Pox

This is a vesicular and pustular disease characterized by eruptions of the skin. A virus is the cause which is easily transmitted from animal to animal. Infected milkers should be isolated and milked last. The disease is more prevalent in colored and black goats who seem to need more copper then the others.

Signs and Symptoms

The main symptoms are pimples that turn into watery blisters, then to sticky and encrusted scabs (like Chicken Pox) on the udder or other hairless areas. The incubation period is from 4 to 7 days. There may be a early transient fever but this can go unnoticed. The udder and teats show sensitivity to touch and may be redder and hotter than usual in the early stages. The lesions are usually confined to the teats and skin of the udder and progress through the recognized stages of papule, vesicle, pustule and scab formation. The papular stage lasts about 2 days and the following vesicular stage appears about the third or fourth day.

The vesicles contain straw colored fluid. This becomes pustular on the eighth day and is followed by the scab or healing stage. The period of time from the appearance of a papule to the healing scab stage is about 8 days.

Herbal Treatment

A short fast followed by a laxative diet of a green nature. Internal dosing with garlic.

Externally wash the area with a lotion of Calendula and Hypericum or Elder flowers and leaves brewed with garlic. Pat Coleby says this condition strikes only when the Goat is deficient in copper. An exterior treatment is a copper and cider vinegar wash which helps the scabs dry up and drop off. Give a copper supplement internally. To make the wash mix a tablespoon of Copper Sulphate with the same amount of Vinegar and mix with 500mls of water this can then be administered with a garden spray bottle and the scabs should start to dry up and drop off.

Homoeopathic treatment

Although this disease is fairly mild the use of the following remedies may cut short the infective process and prevent secondary infections.

Antimonium Crud 6C - This remedy is associated with typical papular and pustular skin lesions especially with a generally dry skin. Signs of indigestion may be present. Dose 3 times daily for 3 days.

Cuprum Aceticum 6C - A leading remedy for pox like eruptions frequently accompanied by cramps and spasms of groups of muscles. Diarrhea may also be present. Dose 3 times daily for 3 days.

Kali Bich 30C - The pustules assume a crater like form with yellowish discharge. Dose 2 times daily for 5 days.

Variolinum 30C - This nosode will be found of values either by its self or used in conjunction with the mentioned remedies. Dose daily for 3 days.

Ranunculus Bulbosus 6C - Another useful remedy for the vesicular stage especially if more prominent on the udder. Dose 3 times daily for 5 days.

Herbal Overview Of The Skin

Conditions such as wounds, burns, bites, ringworm, ticks etc. are all dealt with in First Aid For Animals which gives detailed treatment for these conditions. For problems such as Lumpy Wool look to the Anti-Fungal and Anti Biotic herbs, also consider lotions such as Calendula with Garlic and Tea Tree oil in a spray bottle so as to soak a area and for easy application. For the long drawn out chronic diseases of the skin use the Alteratives especially the ones with a strong affinity to the skin such as Sarsaparilla, Burdock, Cleavers and Nettles. The blood cleansers need time to do their work so always consider using them for 3 months as this is the life cycle of the red blood cells so you would of cleaned most of the blood after using them for this time.

Herbal Actions For The Skin

Alterative - Herbs that gradually restore proper

function to the body, they increase health and vitality. They were once known as the blood cleansers.

Herbs - Black Cohosh, Blue Flag, Burdock, Cleavers, Chaparral, Echinacea, Fumitory, Garlic, Nettles, Pau D'Arco ,Sarsaparilla, Sweet Violets, Yellow Dock.

Anti-biotic - Echinacea, Garlic, Myrrh, Pau D' Arco, Tea Tree Oil

Anti-fungal - Marigold, Cats Claw, Pau D' Arco, Myrrh, Sweet Violets.

Anti-inflammatory - Helps the body to combat inflammations. Herbs mentioned under demulcents, emollients and vulneraries will often act in this way especially when they are applied externally.

Herbs - Arnica, Blue Flag, Cats Claw, Chaparral ,Chickweed, Cleavers, Cranesbill, Chamomile, Eyebright, Ginger, Golden Rod, Guaiacum, Licorice, Marshmallow, Marigold, Pau D' Arco, St Johns Wort, Sweet Violets, Witch Hazel.

Astringent - Contracts tissue which in turn reduces discharges, these herbs contain tannins.

Herbs - Agrimony, Bear Berry, Cranesbill, Chaparral, Chickweed, Comfrey, Eyebright, Golden Rod, Hops, Horsetail, Ladys Mantle, Marigold, Marshmallow, Meadowsweet, Myrrh, Nettles, Raspberry, Sage, Rosemary, Slippery Elm, Shepherds Purse, St Johns Wort, Slippery Elm, Thyme, Witch Hazel, Yarrow.

Emollient - Soothing to the skin. Acts externally the way demulcents do internally.

Herbs - Chickweed, Coltsfoot, Comfrey, Fenugreek, Licorice, Marshmallow, Mullein, Plantain, Slippery Elm.

Parasiticide - Kills parasites and insects.

Herbs - Aniseed, Rosemary,

Vulnerary - Applied externally and aid the body in the healing of wounds and cuts

Herbs - Arnica, Burdock, Chickweed, Comfrey, Cranesbill, Elder, Fenugreek, Garlic, Horsetail, Hyssop, Marigolds, Marshmallow, Mullein, Myrrh, Plantain, Shepherds Purse, Slippery Elm, St Johns Wort, Thyme, Witch Hazel, Yarrow

The Reproductive System

Pregnancy

Herbal Treatment

In kid goat should have access to lots of fresh water and should be left to free range so they can keep fit and slim, this should keep the embryo small and muscular and easy to deliver when the time comes. Heavy feeding should follow after the birth for a high milk yield. Root crops should follow after the goats have birthed with carrots and turnips being especially good, also think of oats for a heavy milk yield rich in fat. Always give roughage with root crops as dry feeds fed with roots prevent digestive problems. Herbs to think of to increase the milk are Marjoram, Sage, Fenugreek, Aniseed, Fennel and Speedwell. Raspberry leaf is the most important herbal aid to a easy birth and should be given to all the breeders especially the ones that have difficult births. All ewes should be given along drink of tepid water after birthing so as to replace the fluids lost from birthing and the giving of milk straight after birth.

Homoeopathic Treatment

The gestation period is around 5 months. Two remedies are important to consider for the maintenance of a healthy pregnancy.

Viburnum Opulis - A remedy for use in the early stages of pregnancy up to one month to 6 weeks. Helps to eliminate the tendency to early miscarriage. Give 30C three times per week for 4 weeks.

Caulophyllum - This remedy is used for the latter stages. Helps to ensure a trouble free birth and tones up the uterus for easy expulsion of the afterbirth. Give 30C three times per week for the last 4 weeks. If the last stage of labor is delayed or weak this remedy should be given again to help speed up normal contractions.

Arnica 30C - This can be used at the time of birthing and given for a few days after as it will help with the bruising and swelling and is good for shock. Give 3 times a day.

BellisPerennis 30C - If the birthing was prolonged or severe give this remedy along with Arnica.

Post Birth Problems
Retained Placenta

If you have a small flock it is a good idea to have some sort of sick bay for animals. I used to have a area for birthing and one of the most important reasons for this is that you would always know if the afterbirth had been expelled. The first thing you should do is to get the kid to suckle as this is the main trigger to release the after birth.

Herbal Treatment - Juliette de Bairacli Levy recommends to keep fasting the doe and then give a strong brew of raspberry leaf and linseed oil strengthened with honey or molasses. All of these substances are stimulating and tonic to the womb. Feverfew can be added to the brew at one to one with the raspberry. Another herb to think of is Pennyroyal which is virtually the specific for this condition.

Homoeopathic Treatment

Homoeopathic remedies to consider are Sepia 30C, Pulsatilla 6c, Satilla 6C and Pyrogen 1M.

Sabina - Useful when the condition is associated with the retention of the afterbirth or miscarriage especially in those cases showing blood stained discharges. Give 6C every hour for 6 doses.

Hemorrhage

Herbal Treatment

Astringents are the main herbs that you use to stop bleeding. Two of the strongest ones are Shepherds Purse and Cranesbill. Make a 1 to 10 lotion of either of these herbs and if bleeding cannot be controlled use a small syringe without the needle to gently inject into the womb, hopefully this will spasm the ends of the bleeding vessels and stop the flow of blood.

Homoeopathic Treatment

This does not occur to often but when it does try to match one of the remedies below.

Ipecacuanah 6C - Blood accumulates in the uterus and is then expelled in a bright red flood. Give every hour for 5 doses.

Crotalus 1M - If the blood comes away as a steady drip. Give every hour for 4 doses.

Hammamelis 30C - Dark blood indicating a venous origin will need this remedy. Give 1 dose every 2 hours up to 5 times.

Secale 30C - Very stringy blood indicates this remedy.

Give 1 dose every 2 hours up to 5 times.

Metritis Acute

Metritis or inflammation of the womb can be acute or chronic. The acute condition is associated with the birth and is usually a bacterial invasion of the lining of the womb. Chief among the causes of this condition is the retained placenta together with infection which gains entrance to the genital tract.

Signs and Symptoms

This usually occurs 24 hours after kidding. There is a rise in temperature followed by a loss of appetite and the Doe is uneasy and lethargic. Respirations are increased and there may be a expression of anxiety on the face, abdominal pains, coma. The vulva and vagina may be inflamed and dark red. Discharge is not always present but if it is it may vary from a yellowish color through to blood stained.

Herbal Treatment

We will start off by telling you how this problem on the pregnancy side could of probably been avoided in the first place. If the Doe was given the herbs Raspberry or Squaw Vine in the last months of pregnancy these herbs would of toned and strengthened the uterus and the problem may of been avoided. At the onset of labor if the herb Golden Seal was used it could of given the Doe the extra strength and energy to have a successful and problem free labor, this usually works by making the contractions stronger. When the kids are born it is usually when they start to suckle that triggers the expulsion of the placenta. Inflammations of the uterus arising from infection should be treated with the main immune boosting herbs mainly Echinacea, Garlic and another good one if you have got it is Myrrh. To these herbs consider adding Ladys Mantle (astringent) Black or Blue Cohosh, or Saw Palmetto. Cleavers could be used as a Alterative for cleaning out the system. A lotion of Calendula could be used to clean the outside area especially if it is red and sore also think of adding Hypericum to the lotion for pain relief.

Juliette de Bairacli Levy recommends to fast the Doe for 2 days followed by a milk and molasses mono diet. Dose with garlic night and morning and give Licorice juice in milk twice daily. Keep the Doe warm. Give a internal douche with a brew of lavender. If there was bleeding I would consider adding Ladys Mantle or shepherds purse to the douche. Calendula is another herb to think of adding.

Homoeopathic Treatment

Treatment should be started as bad signs start to appear after parturition especially after dead kids and a difficult labor.

Aconitum 1M - Should be given at once so as to quickly allay shock, fear and anxiety and regulate the circulation. Give every hour for 4 hours.

Belladonna 1M - Indicated when the animal is hot to touch with a full bounding pulse and dilated pupils. Signs of cerebral excitement may be present with extreme cases convulsions. Give every hour for 5 hours.

Lillum Tig 30C - A good general remedy for uterine congestion leading to blood stained discharges and straining in the pelvic region.

Secale 30C- Hemorrhages are present when this remedy is considered, the blood is fluid and dark, the patient is cadaverous looking with cold extremities which are deficient in blood supply. Give twice daily for 10 days.

Sabina 6C- Useful when the condition is associated with the retention of the afterbirth or miscarriage especially in those cases showing blood stained discharges. Give every hour for 6 doses.

Pyrogen 1M - This nosode is indicated when a weak thready pulse alternates with a high temperature or vice versa. The most useful remedy in septic conditions. Give every 2 hours for 4 doses.

Mastitis

The cause can be a combination of factors such as faulty management, exposure to cold winds and wet weather, injuries from blows and sharp objects, insufficient stripping of the udder in milking and bacterial infections caught from others or as a result of poor hygiene. Mastitis can occur anytime during lactation but is frequently seen after birth.

Signs and Symptoms

The disease may begin with attacks of shivering and general unease in the animal. Appetite fails and fever develops. Sometimes the temperature rises as high as

104 or 105 degrees with high fever being a typical symptom of the ailment. The entire udder rapidly hardens and becomes very hot to the touch. General signs include changes in milk secretion resulting in abnormalities such as clots and changes in the size and consistency of the udder quarters involved. There is frequently also a systemic reaction. Sometime the Doe tries to keep the legs from contacting the udder and as a result may walk with a different gait and stand with the rear legs apart. The acute form frequently comes after birth and a less severe form sometimes at drying off. The onset is usually sudden and can be recognized by swelling of the gland and changes in the milk. The swelling may take several forms ranging from slight edema to a hot painful enlargement. This condition can happen at any time during lactation. Isolate the effected Ewe.

Herbal Treatment

The Doe must be confined indoors for the treatment in a well-ventilated area. For the really stubborn cases begin with a cleansing fast of 2 days with water only allowed or water and a solution of molasses with a purge given in the evening. A effective purge is 2 ounces of Epsoms Salts, one ounce of linseed oil, half a teaspoonful of ground ginger, one teaspoonful of grated Gentian root and 2 ounces of warm water, give mixed in oatmeal gruel to make 1 and a half pints. Garlic is the main herb to be given at the dosage of 1 whole root grated into one cup of water with half a cup given morning and night. Wood Sage (has a affinity to the udder) was also given with this treatment but is now very difficult to find. Wood Sage can be made into a lotion and applied to the udder.

Humans sometimes use a cabbage leaf poultice for this condition, get some cabbage leafs and pound them so they are bruised all over and apply to the affected area, I will leave you to figure out how to do this as I aren't all that sure myself as usually women use a oversized bra to hold the leaves in place. Photolacca tincture in small doses is the main herb for mastitis though I believe the Homoeopathic potency is far better and faster acting then the tincture. To the Homoeopathic Dose you could make a lotion for external application of Photolacca but make it a very mild lotion as this is a strong remedy so make it about 1 to 20 in strength. The main immune boosting herbs should also be used these are Echinacea, Garlic and Myrrh as well as the alteratives such as Cleavers.

Pat Coleby says Goats with mastitis should be given a extra teaspoon of dolomite and the same of Vitamin C night and morning until the infection clears.

Juliette de Bairacli Levy recommends that the kid should be allowed to suckle as the milk can be kept healthy by feeding large garlic balls or garlic tablets to the mother twice a day because the garlic crosses over to the milk.

Homoeopathic Treatment.

A wise farmer would treat this on a herd basis by determining which bacteria is the cause and then making a Nosode (potency made from a disease product) of that bacteria to the 30C potency and treating the herd with it by dosing the animals water troughs.

Common frequent remedies used on a individual basis are as below.

Aconite 6X - This should be used as routine in all acute cases especially in those that develop suddenly, it will allay tension and restlessness, cause may be from exposure from cold dry winds. Dose every half hour for 6 doses.

Arnica 30C - Indicated when mastitis develops as a result of injury to the mammary tissue, blood may be present in the milk. Dose 3 times daily for 3 days.

Apis 6C - This is a useful remedy for freshly birthed Does showing edema of the udder and surrounding tissues. The mammary vein is usually engorged in this case. Dose every 3 hours for 4 doses.

Belladonna 1M - Indicated usually in the acute form post-partum. The udder shows acute swelling and redness, pain is obvious on touch, the animal will feel hot with full bounding pulse. Dose every hour for 4 doses.

Bryonia 30C - Indicated where the udder swelling is hard and indurated. In acute cases pain will be relieved by pressure on the udder and such cases are frequently presented with the animal lying down as this appears to give relief. Chronic forms showing fibrosis should benefit from this remedy. Dose 4 hourly for 4 doses while in the chronic form dose twice weekly for a month.

Phytolacca 30C - A useful remedy for both acute and

chronic cases. Acute form may show curdled milk and clots while in the latter small clots may appear in mid lactation. This is probably the most useful remedy for the average chronic case. Dose 3 times daily for 3 days followed once daily for 4 days.

Urtica Urens 6X - For acute forms showing edema which may be in the form of plaques frequently extending to the perineal area. Dose every hour for 4 doses.

Hepar Sulph 6X - This low potency will help promote suppuration and clearing of the udder contents in cases of C. Pyogenes or summer mastitis infection. Dose every 3 hours for 4 doses. Once the udder has been cleared of purulent material a dose or 2 of a higher potency should be given to complete the cure.

Ip[ecac 30C - This is a useful remedy for controlling intra-mammary bleeding which results in pink milk. Dose 3 times daily for 3 days.

Milk Fever

This is one of the lactation diseases that can be seen in Goats which have attained there highest productive period or can arise just after kidding. The immediate cause is a reduction or fall in the level of calcium in the system. This is brought about by to little calcium in the diet together with the demands made on the dams reserves by the developing foetus and finally by the onset of lactation.

Signs and Symptoms

The average attack takes place within 72 hours of

birth but some cases can occur a little latter after the onset of lactation. The onset of the attack is often sudden. Preliminary signs include trembling, muscle spasms and restlessness with these becoming more severe until the animal becomes wobbly and finally collapses. Coma may or may not set in but when it does a common pose is that of the animal lying recumbent with the head turned around to one side resting on the neck. If the neck is straightened forcibly the head upon release returns to its former position. Just as frequent is the patient laying stretched out and groaning. Muscular tremors may be seen. Tympany sets in if the animal has collapsed with the rumen uppermost. There is more or less complete bowel stasis leading to bloat if the Goat is lying on its side. Congestion of the eye is usually present and the breathing labored along with a soft and slow pulse. The body temperature is usually below normal not high as milk fever would suggest.

Treatment

The classical treatment of this disease is by intra venous or subcutaneous injection of calcium and allied salts and in the great majority of cases this is successful with no other treatment being needed.

Homoeopathic Treatment

The following remedies will greatly reduce the risk of relapse and help prevent complications of the nervous system.

Belladonna 1M - This is indicated when the animal is excitable or violent, throwing its head about, with staring pupils and congested eyes. Dose every half hour for 4 doses.

Mag Phos 6C - Should always be given as a routine to help elevate a deficiency being brought on by the lack of calcium. Dose every half hour for 4 doses.

Stramonium 200C - When nervous symptoms are more often seen on peripheral parts with less brain involvement. Twitches are commonly seen. Dose every hour for 6 doses.

Thyroid 3X - This remedy will help regulate thyroid function as this gland is deeply involved in the disease process. Dose every hour for 3 doses followed by one 3 times daily for 2 days.

Cuprum Met 1M - This remedy will assist in relieving muscular cramping when the animal is on the way to recovery. Dose twice daily for 2 days.

Colchicum 200C - If rumenal bloat is a problem give this remedy every half hour for 4 doses.

Teats Sore Or Damaged

The delicate tissues of the teat sometimes become chapped and develop deep fissures.

Symptoms - The Doe will not tolerate the lamb feeding.

Herbal Treatment - Juliette de Bairacli Levy recommends to treat alternately with warm almond oil as a salve and bathed with a brew of equal parts elder blossom and marshmallow. Raw cucumber juice has been effective. I would use Calendula and Hypericum Lotion (1 to 10) as this is a great healer of all wounds and also helps to relieve the pain.

Herbal Overview Of The Reproductive System

Below are some of the actions to consider for this system. In the Astringents the herbs underlined are the best to use to stop bleeding. Use the Alteratives for Chronic diseases of this system and maybe add some of the Emmenagogues to them after reading up on the individual herbs and adding the one that works in the direction you want.

Herbal Actions For The Reproductive System

Alterative - Herbs that gradually restore proper function to the body, they increase health and vitality. They were once known as the blood cleansers.

Herbs - Black Cohosh, Dong Quai, Damiana, Skullcap.

Anti-biotic - Chaparral, Echinacea, Garlic, Myrrh, Pau D' Arco, Reshi.

Anti-fungal - Marigold, Cats Claw, Pau D' Arco, Myrrh, Sweet Violets.

Anti-inflammatory - Helps the body to combat inflammations. Herbs mentioned under demulcents, emollients and vulnerary's will often act in this way especially when they are applied externally.

Herbs - Cranesbill, Chamomile, Eyebright, Feverfew, Ginger, Golden Rod, Ladys Mantle,

Licorice, Marshmallow, Meadowsweet, Marigold, Pau D' Arco, St Johns Wort, Witch Hazel.

Anti-Tumor - Burdock, Cleavers, Reshi, Shitake, Sweet Violets.

Antispasmodic - Prevents or eases spasms and cramps.

Herbs - Aniseed, Angelica, Black Cohosh, Chamomile, Fennel, Hyssop, Motherwort, Rosemary, Rue, Sage, Skullcap, St Johns Wort, Thyme, Valerian, Vervain.

Anti-viral - Astragalus, Cats claw, Echinacea, Garlic, Myrrh?, Shitake, St Johns Wort, Pau D'Arco.

Astringent - Contracts tissue which in turn reduces discharges, these herbs contain tannins.

Herbs - Agrimony, Cranesbill, Eyebright, Golden Rod, Ladys Mantle, Marigold, Raspberry, Shepherds Purse, St Johns Wort, Witch Hazel.

Emmenagogue - Stimulates and normalizes the menstrual flow, tonics for the female reproductive system.

Herbs - Black Cohosh, Chamomile, Fenugreek, Gentian, Ginger, Juniper, Ladys Mantle, Marigold, Motherwort, Parsley, Penny Royal, Peppermint, Parsley, Raspberry, Sage, Rosemary, Rue, Shepherds Purse, St Johns Wort, Tansy, Thyme, Valerian, Vervain, Wormwood, Yarrow.

Galactagogue - Helps increase the flow of milk in females.

Herbs - Aniseed, Fennel, Fenugreek, Milk Thistle,

Raspberry, Vervain.

NOTES

Disease Conditions

Coccidiosis

This is an important protozoal disease affecting many housed Goats although it can occur under other conditions. It is caused by various species of the Eimeria family which parasite the intestinal canal producing what are known as oocysts which pass out in the droppings and after undergoing a definite life cycle are then ready to effect other Goats on ingestion of the affected material. Spread of infection is through contamination of water and food supply. Treatment is usually with drugs such as Sulphadimidine and a thorough cleaning of living area and water vessels

Signs and Symptoms

Various forms of virulence are recognized ranging from mild to hyperacute. Mild forms show little more than loose stools with blood being absent. The more acute form presents as a blood stained or bloody diarrhea accompanied by severe straining. Dehydration normally occurs. The hyperacute form may yield little or no symptoms with the animal dying a few hours after the ingestion of the oocysts. Symptoms for kids may appear as persistent scouring which may be blood tinged, loss of appetite leading to loss of condition, dull stiff coat, rapid breathing.

In older animals the condition can become chronic and is often unsuspected though milk production will be down and occasionally diarrhea with a foetid smell develops.

Herbal Treatment

Garlic aided by molasses is the great specific for worms or other parasites. One large or 2 small plants can be chopped finely and mixed well with flower and black treacle and rolled into balls the size of walnuts. Flaked garlic root can also be used to make balls. Give 2 to 3 balls a day. For better results give while fasting. Food additions of raw grated carrot, raw desiccated coconut and seeds of pumpkins, papaya, grapes and melon are all worm removing likewise with raw grated radish and turnip. Pat Coleby says he had no more problems with this condition after he planted some Mallow (Malva Plants) in the paddock which he says have a reputation of preventing this condition and also noticed that the stock which had the right amount of Copper supplemented seemed not to get the disease.

Homoeopathic Treatment

Aconitum 1M - If seen in the early stages this remedy may help limit the disease process. Dose once every half hour for 4 doses.

Arsenicum Alb 1M - This remedy should prove effective in the milder case showing diarrhea and loss of condition with a dry coat. Dose 3 times daily for 4 days.

Ipecac 30C - A good anti-hemorrhagic remedy that appears to have a specific action on the intestine in the presence of protozoa. Dose 3 times daily for 5 days.

Mercurius Corr 200C - This remedy is valuable where

there is severe straining accompanied by dysenteric slimy stools. Dose 2 times daily for 5 days.

China 6C - This remedy will help restore strength after loss of body fluid following diarrhoea. Dose 3 times per day for 3 days.

Veratrum Alb 30C - This remedy should help milder cases showing persistent diarrhoea of a explosive type with threatened collapse. Dose 3 times daily for 5 days.

Clostridial Infections

Enterotoxaemia

Can also be known as Pulpy kidney disease (Autopsy often shows soft spots on the kidneys) and overeating disease. This condition is associated with bacteria of the clostridial (type D effecting Goats and Sheep) family and causes a serious intestinal disease especially in young kids often resulting in death. It is caused by a Bacterium that is always present but when in large amounts and deprived of oxygen in the digestive system it produces toxins that are absorbed into the blood. The proper conditions for this can be produced by overfeeding. Goats can build up resistance to the poison in small regular amounts but they can't handle sudden surges. Causes can be sudden changes in diet like moving from a poor paddock to one of lush crops or pasture, overfeeding of grains or concentrates. The best prevention is proper feeding on a suitable bulky fibrous diet and there is also a vaccine for this condition.

Signs and Symptoms

Systemic symptoms soon appear after exposure to infection resulting in high temperature, severe diarrhea usually of a peculiarly evil smell and loss of appetite. With some strains there may be bloat or staggering. In the very acute form the disease progresses rapidly and the Goat may die within 2 hours. The Goat may stagger, twitch, convulse (have fits) and show signs of shock before death. In the more common acute form it may take 24 hours for the Goat to die and they appear dull and stagger and may convulse. Diarrhea is the first symptom usually yellowish green which may change latter to a gelatinous whitish mucous latter having blood through it. Finally large clots of blood and sheets of bowel lining appear. By this time the animal is shivering and cold to the touch. This is best felt in the mouth, the temp may drop to 33 degrees. Latter the animal lays down struggles violently cries pitifully and dies soon after. Often animals with acute symptoms are found dead in the morning.

Herbal Treatment

A lot of texts say there is no treatment for this condition but I don't give up that easy. It seem obvious that if it is the toxins that kill then we must get rid of these as fast as possible so I would be inclined to start off with a good purge so as to clear the toxins from the system so go to the Digestive System Section and see what it says there paying special attention to Slippery Elm especially in the young animals. Pat Coleby has treated successfully animals with this condition so I shall write down word for word the treatment he used.

Initial treatment is 250 ml of warm cooking oil. this always seems to be beneficial in any case of bad scouring. Give 20cc of Vitamin C, with 2cc of vitamin B12 and 2 mls of VAM by injection in the same syringe. Then give 2 teaspoonfuls of ascorbic acid powder orally followed by a large teaspoon of each of the following, dolomite, slippery elm powder and crushed Garlic tablets. Repeat all except the oil, B12 and VAM at 2 hourly Intervals.

Homoeopathic Treatment

Pyrogen 1M - May give relief in mild cases ,septic inflammations with offensive discharges, is needed when there is a discrepancy between pulse and temperature eg raised temperature alternating with a weak and thready pulse and vice versa.

Arsenic Alb 1M - May give some relief in mild cases, may be needed when stools are dark and blood stained, the animal is restless and there is a thirst for small quantities of water.

Note - See related conditions in The Digestive System

Tetanus (Lock Jaw)

This disease is caused by the bacterium Clostridium tetani gaining entrance to the body through puncture or other deep wounds that are not exposed to the air. It can be common in goats following castration.

Symptoms - The animal walks in a unsteady manner, there is muscle stiffness and muscular spasms. Severe cases involve the central nervous system with convulsions and death from respiratory failure.

Herbal Treatment

The main herb to think of here is Hypericum also known as St Johns Wort. This herb is used as a nervine anti-viral and bacterial. Traditionally it has been used to help prevent tetanus especially in horses that have trodden on a nail that has gone through the fetlock. The treatment for horses was to pour straight tincture into the wound in the hope it would kill the bacteria. Treat all wounds with Hypericum and Calendula tinctures mixed half and half diluted with water. See the Animal First Aid Book.

Homoeopathic Treatment

The following remedies may give some relief and in mild cases may lead to cure especially if started early.

Acconitum - For the fear and anxiety which lambs may display, always give at the first signs of a problem. Give 10M every hour for 4 doses.

Curare - Helps where muscle stiffness is prominent. Give 30c three times daily for 7days.

Strychninum - The arching of the back together with extension of limbs and head matches the symptoms of this remedy. Give 200c twice daily for 3 days.

Hypericum - This remedy may help in limiting the spread of the toxin. Give 1M three times daily for 7 days.

Ledum - This is the main remedy for puncture wounds especially if they feel cold. Give frequently in the 6C potency.

Tetanus Nosode - Combine the nosode with the selected remedy. Use for 7 days in the 30th potency.

Other Clostridial Infections

Clostridial bacteria can be found in the soil where they can survive for a long time. Most also occur quite naturally in the gut and manure of animals. The Clostridial bacteria grow only where there is little oxygen such as in rotting vegetable matter in the soil or in dead or bruised tissue inside the body of a animal. In the body the bacteria produces powerful and fatal toxins.

Black Disease - I've taken this from the sheep book as this condition may effect goats. This condition is associated with liver damage primarily caused by liver fluke. Here the strain is Clostridial oedematiens type B and spores of this can be found in the soil and livers of sheep on the farms where the disease occurs. Other signs can be dark skin, the wool plucks out, sudden death and a rapid decomposition. This bacteria thrives in areas of liver necrosis caused by the migration of liver flukes and then produces a powerful necrotizing toxin. The disease is worldwide especially in places where fluke and sheep meet.

Symptoms - Most cases occur in summer and early fall when liver fluke infection is at its height. The disease is most prevalent in 1 to 4 year old sheep and is limited to animals infected with liver flukes. Rapid onset of dullness, followed by a unsteady gate then an inability to move. There is collapse and quiet death within a few hours.

Prevention - Vaccinate and treat for fluke.

Black Leg - Caused by Clostridial chauvoei and commonly follows bruising during handling, shearing, docking, birthing and castration. Spores of C.chauvoei survive well in the soil and in sheep the majority of cases arise from contamination of the wound.

Symptoms - Within 48 hours there is a high fever and if muscles are involved the animal becomes stiff and unwilling to move. There can be skin discoloration, swelling at the wound site, edema under the skin and gas production may be present. In cases of gangrenous metritis after birth death soon follows after a period of profound prostration. Again here there is rapid decomposition after death.

Prevention - Vaccinate and practice good hygiene. Use Calendula lotion on all wounds, if concerned make lotion stronger.

Malignant Oedema (blood poisoning, Gas Gangrene) - This is caused by the infection of the wound by or up to 4 different strains of Clostridial bacteria. The condition occurs as a result of the

wound becoming contaminated with soil which has spores of bacteria in it.

Symptoms - Signs appear rapidly after infection and at the site of the infection a swelling will develop which will pit on pressure. Gas may be detected as the skins darkens and becomes tensor. A high fever develops and toxemia develops. The animal dies with in one to two days.

Prevention - Vaccinate and practice good hygiene. Use Calendula lotion on all wounds, if concerned make lotion stronger.

Braxy - Caused by C.septicum and appears in late autumn and early winter. Usually effects kids born in the previous spring as older animals appear to develop some type of immunity to the disease. The disease appears to be triggered by the ingestion of frosted food

Symptoms - Disease is of sudden and short duration with animals suffering high fever, depression and anorexia. There can be abdominal pain together with the accumulation of abdominal gas. Recumbency and coma are followed by death within a few hours of the onset of the disease.

Herbal Overview For Clostridial Infections

You would be lucky if your animal survives but here is what we can try and it will give you an idea for similar problems. If the problems in the digestive system give a strong purge immediately use Castor oil as this is a strong purgative and speed is of the essence as we need to get the bacteria making the toxins out fast or the toxins will kill. If the problem comes from a wound use a knife and re open the wound and clean with Calendula and Hypericum lotion. In all cases give a large dose of Echinacea and Garlic. Echinacea is used to fight blood borne toxins especially from bacteria as well as boost the immune system while the Garlic is a strong antibacterial. Use Hypericum internally in tetanus as well as on the wound. This condition would suit the herb Astragalus which is a immune boosting herb that is mainly used in chronic diseases but the main reason we are using it is that it can put oxygen in the system which may upset this bacteria as it does not like oxygen.

Pink Eye

This is a Rickettsial disease seen mainly in the summer months affecting Goats kept in unhygienic conditions, but also outside in fields and wooded surroundings. The pathogen gains entry after damage has been done to the eye like a little scratch; the trouble is most often seen in dry, dusty and windy weather where the eye may get scratched. The disease is highly contagious and can be spread by flies. The disease has a incubation period of a week.

Signs and Symptoms

The condition may attack one or both eyes, the eyes start to water and the conjunctiva becomes red and inflamed and the eyelids swell. If treatment is commenced quickly the condition may not pass this point. A white spot develops on the cornea leading eventually to a opaque covering and ulceration. Secondary infections by bacteria can be common and leads to the development of ophthalmia with resulting purulent discharges. The Goat may go blind (but may recover sight), loose condition, reduced milk yield and look miserable. One must appreciate the pain of a badly damaged eye. If no action is taken the whole eye becomes blood shot and may rupture causing permanent blindness.

Herbal Treatment

Equal parts of the tinctures of Calendula, Hypercum and Euphrasia (Eye Bright) mixed together and bottled. From this bottle we will now make a lotion at a strength of 1 to 10. We will now use this lotion to wipe and clean the eyes with. Use cotton wool balls to apply the lotion but use a different one for each Goat. This should be done at least 4 times a day, I would be inclined to do it every 2 hours. Internally I would give Cod Liver Oil (Vitamins A and D) and would think about giving Echinacea so as to build up the immune system along with Garlic which would help fight the infection. Pat Coleby treats this condition by filling a 10ml syringe with Cod Liver Oil and squirts 2ml into the affected eye and the rest down the throat. He says the topical application is very effective. Another remedy he uses for removing the soreness is crushing a Bio-Chemic Cell Salt tablet of Ferrum Phos to powder and gently blowing it into the open eye. He says the disease is caused by a Vitamin A deficiency in the animals.

Homoeopathic Treatment

Aconitum 1M - This remedy should be given early, the animal at this stage may be listless with a slightly inflamed eye. Dose once every hour for 4 doses.

Argentum Nit 30C - If ophthalmia is threatening with purulent discharges beginning use this remedy. Dose 3 times daily for 4 days.

Acid Nitric 200C - If corneal ulceration has developed this remedy may help. Dose once daily for 10 days.

Euphrasia 12C - Red sore looking eyes, best used at the beginning maybe after Acconitum.
Dose about 5 times a day

Silica 200c - This is the remedy of choice once corneal opacity has developed. It will hasten the absorption of the scar tissue. Dose 3 times per week for 3 weeks.

Caseous Lymphadenitis (Cheesy Gland)

This is a chronic condition which is capable of spreading from one Goat to another. It is characterized by multiple abscesses which appear in the lymph glands. All age groups can be affected but it is more likely to be encountered in the older age groups. The causative organism is Corynebabcterium Ovis which usually gains entry through a wound.

Incubation period is relatively long up to 4 months in some cases.

Signs and Symptoms

Swellings appear in the lymph nodes with the main sites being under the jaw and parotid glands, other sites which may become affected are the supramammary and the popliteal. Most of the cervical lymph nodes can be affected in severe outbreaks. Rapid breathing and coughing are signs that deeper lymph nodes are effected. The abscess starts as a flat hardening at the back of the jaw, developing into a boil varying from the size of a twenty cent piece to that of a tennis ball depending on the Goats immunity. Abscesses as they mature become hairless and upon maturation yield a pus which is yellowish and sometimes greenish.

Herbal Treatment

Hot poultices are very effective at drawing the core out of boils so here we shall use a hot poultice of slippery elm (half a tea spoon full) with about 4 drops of castor oil which is also good at drawing out unwanted matter, mix this with a bit of boiling water to form a hot paste.

Apply to the area and leave on for 20 minutes and repeat several times till suppuration occurs. After suppuration you can mix together a bit of calendula and comfrey creams and apply them to the area. These two herbs working together will speed up the healing time, disinfect and reduce or prevent scaring. Internally think of Echinacea to build immunity,

Garlic for its antibiotic effect and to this we can add a few lymphatic herbs such as Fenugreek which promotes lymphatic drainage and maybe Poke Root but only in very small doses as this is a powerful lymphatic cleanser.

Homoeopathic Treatment

There are many useful remedies to consider in controlling the spread of this infection and limiting it within the affected animal. These Include-

Silicea 200C - This is probably the most important remedy being well proven in the treatment of chronic cold abscesses. Dose 3 times per week for 4 weeks.

Calc Fluor 30C - The hardness and swelling of the lymph nodes which develop during abscess formation will be aided by this remedy. Dose once daily for ten days.

Gunpowder 6C - This remedy has proved useful in the treatment of multiple abscesses and is beneficial in the early stages of abscess formation. Dose 3 times daily for 5 days.

Tarentula Cubensis 30C - Excessive hardness surrounding the abscess with a tendency to necrosis of skin calls for this remedy. Dose 3 times daily for 5 days.

Phosphorus 200C - If the supramammary lymph nodes are more prominently affected then others this remedy may help. Dose 3 times per week for 4 weeks.

Merc Sol 30C - If the pus is greenish this is a keynote for this remedy. It should benefit the submaxillary and parotid glands in particular. Dose once daily for 7 days.

C. Ovis Nosode 30C - This can be prepared from the pus of any gland and after potentising given daily for 7 days and can be combined with any selected remedy. The nosode should be considered as a prophylactic measure in all flocks which are at risk. A twice monthly dose should be given for 4 months.

Johne's Disease

This chronic wasting disease is also known as Paratuberculosis affects cattle, sheep, goats and most ruminants. This disease is associated with the gradual loss of weight following the infection of the intestinal mucosa by a bacillus known as Mycobacterium Johnei. It is prevalent worldwide. There is a long incubation period sometimes with the infection showing 18 months later.

Symptoms - This disease is a long term chronic contagious enteritis. Emaciation develops gradually, bowel movements appear to be soft and milk production can be affected. The disease is characterized by weight loss and diarrhea, the diarrhea is intermittent and is typically thick and does not contain any blood or mucous and is passed without much problems. Over weeks or months the diarrhea becomes more severe and there is further weight loss and the coat color may fade. In dairy cattle the milk yield falls. Animals remain alert and the temperature and appetite remain normal though thirst may be increased. The disease is progressive and ends in emaciation and death. In advanced cases sheep may shed wool easily.

Herbal Treatment

Concentrate on the antibacterials especially Garlic and give Echinacea to build up the immune system. After a month replace the Echinacea with Astragalus which is the immune booster for chronic diseases.

Homoeopathic Treatment

This is hard to treat and there is often relapses. Give the nosode of this disease on a flock basis, dose each animal twice weekly for 6 weeks. This may help build up a measure of protection.

Acid Nit - This remedy has helped some cases of colitis and may control the condition by restoring tone to the intestinal mucosa. Give 200C three times per week for 4 weeks.

Aloe - There may be signs of pain and rectal irritation if this remedy is indicated. Stools are blood stained and contain mucous. Give 30C daily for 14 days.

Gaertner - The use of this bowel nosode is indicated in the younger animal, it has a stimulating effect on the bowel mucosa. Give 30C one dose daily for 7 days.

Johne's Disease Nosode - This should add the action of the other remedies and can be given in the 30C for 7 days.

Listeriosis

This bacterial infection affects a wide range of animals

including man and is seen worldwide but in more temperate and colder climates. Grazing animals ingest the organism and recontaminate the soil with their faeces. Sometimes referred as circling disease. This condition is related to the central nervous system and take various forms ranging from inflammation of the brain to acute septicemia and abortion. Listeria that are ingested or inhaled tend to cause septicemia, abortion and latent infection. Those that gain entry through wounds or tissue tend to localize in the intestinal wall, medulla oblongata and placenta or to cause encephalitis. This disease responds to penicillin if given early enough. Silage contaminated with infected soil can spread the disease.

Symptoms - Encephalitis is the most common form of Listeriosis in goats. The patient circles constantly and may show head pain by pressing its head against any convenient object. In the abortion form expulsion of the foetus is confined to the latter stages of pregnancy and may affect 20% of the flock. The course in sheep and goats can be rapid and death may occur in 24 to 48 hours after the onset. The animals don't eat and are depressed and disoriented; they may propel themselves into corners or lean against stationary objects or circle on the effected side. There may be facial paralysis with a drooping ear, flaccid lips and a lowered eyelid on the effected side with almost continuous salivation. Terminally affected animals fall and can't rise and may continue to make running movements.

Herbal Treatment

See Encephalitis in the Nervous System. Herbs may be to slow in working to help with this fast paced disease but it is worth a try for it could slow it down.

Homoeopathic Treatment

Stramonium 200C - If the circling is from right to left when this remedy is indicated. Dose 3 times per week for 4 weeks.

Cicuta Virosa 30C - Circling the opposite way, the head may be bent back. Dose once daily for 10 days.

Sufonal 30C - Signs of pain or distress are seen when the head is moved. The eyes have a blood shot appearance. If made to rise there may be vertigo like movements such as staggering or incoordination. Dose 3 times daily for 5 days.

Listeria Nosode 30C - This should aid the selected remedy and given by itself to the rest of the flock for protection against the disease.

Herbal Supplement

Important Please Read

This Herbal Supplement is composed of herbs used for animals. We are going to concentrate on these Herbs as they are fairly safe. I have left in some of the dosages given to horses as a comparison. At the end of every section in the Cattle book for example The Digestive System there is a Overview of that section listing what are the common herbal actions needed for that system. The reason that is there is to teach you to think in the Actions you require for the treatment of your patient which gives you a more holistic view of the patient and what's happening. This makes you really start to think about what you are doing instead of thinking I will use the herb I used last time. Every case and every being is individual, think of what you are doing and why. Now for the hardest part, be patient, healing takes time. In the Actions explanation for example Demulcent, you will be told the meaning then given a list of herbs that are commonly known to be strong in that action, some will be different from what is listed in this herbal so you will have to do your own research but they should be generally safe for animal use as most of them come out of my Animal Herbal, this allows you a greater selection of herbs to use especially when you can't source the ones mentioned in the treatment section. Nearly all of the herbs mentioned have been historically used for animals and this is my part in making sure they are not forgotten again. I prefer using liquid to medicate in tinctures, extracts or infusion form even though there can be some controversy over the alcohol, the reason for this is that liquid spreads through the intestines a greater distance then the dry form which insures maximum absorption. In the herbal where no doses are mentioned these are the ones that are usually best in extract or tincture form and the manufacturers should give you the dose to match the strength that they have made it in.

Introduction To Herbal Medicine

Herbal Medicine has been in use and developed continuously since the beginning of time. It mainly evolved from observations from what plants did and the affects they had on people along with their animals. There is also what they call the Doctrine of Signatures which works like this, that flower really looks like a eye, maybe it helps sore eyes?. I'll give it a try as my eyes are so sore and red. You know my eye really feels a lot better now, I think I will call that plant Eye Bright (Euphrasia) and tell my friends all about it especially my Dad who gets sore eyes to. In this way hundreds of plants were identified that have a medical action and no doubt there were also a lot of casualties.

The next great leap in herbal medicine was the Roman Empire of 2000 years ago. The Great Armies of Rome all had their own Medical Corps with Doctors, Battle Surgeons and Orderlies. It was these men who already had the knowledge of the Greeks that started to put together the best medical manuals in the world while at the same time started developing and using medical instruments and tools some of which are still used today. As the Romans conquered the known world more medicines and knowledge were found and assimilated.

The next great leap was modern Chemistry which allowed us to see exactly what herbs were made up of and what parts of the herb causes its medical action. Drug companies have made billions of Dollars from this information as they find the main active ingredient and then make a synthetic version of it, one good example that we all know of is Valium which is the synthetic version of the active ingredient from the herb Valerian. Leaving aside the Drug Companies lets see how Chemistry changed the way that modern herbalists think.

Modern science allows us to now know what Actions our herbs perform on the body so we shall carry on using Valerian as a example and see what Medical Actions Valerian has on the body.

The Actions of Valerian are Sedative, Hypnotic (sleep inducing), Anti Spasmodic (stops twitches, cramps etc), Hypotensive (lowers Blood Pressure) and Carminative (calms and relaxes the tummy). Herbalists call Valerian the Herbal Tranquillizer and if you look at the above you can see why for if you can't sleep and your blood pressures up along with a gurgling tummy and a eye constantly twitching you definitely need to be calmed down.

The modern herbalist is trained to think in actions. There are many reasons for this but the main ones are to stop them from just using a handful of their favorite herbs and to train the mind to work in the method of thinking in actions that are needed. If we start thinking in the actions that are needed for a patient it makes us consider the problem in far more depth than just using our favorite herb and it forces our thinking to be far more holistic by taking in consideration the whole of the patient not just the part or the system we wish to treat.

Lets take a look at thinking in actions. The animal has a cough, but when it coughs it can't stop and the cough sounds a bit like whooping cough. The animal also sounds a little hoarse and the temperature is also elevated. The actions that come into mind for this are expectorant for the cough, anti spasmodics for the whooping quality of the cough and demulcents to sooth the sore throat. These are the obvious actions and we can add many more if we wish such as immune boosters for acute diseases, diaphoretics to reduce the temperature and prevent a fever and the list goes on. Next we look at how Herbal Actions are used in making Herbal Formulas.

Another point to make before we go to the formula making is that Professional Herbalists use Herbs in the form of Tinctures (water and alcohol solutions) as this allows them to mix formulas in any proportions that they like and also allows long term storage without spoiling.

Making Herbal Formulas

You should never have more the 5 Herbs in a herbal formula otherwise you start to lose track of what you are doing and how the formula is changing the symptoms. Always try to keep things simple. One of the herbs in the formula is used to force the formula into the body, to keep it simple we will only use three, they are Licorice, Ginger and Cayenne.

As an example let's use an animal with a cough. After further study of the case we decide that this is a Acute Disease for it came on quick and is fast acting not slow like a Chronic Disease. Listening to the animals cough we decide that it is a dry cough and upon looking at the animals nose we can't see any mucus. Let's list the actions to consider.

Expectorants - Licorice, Aniseed, Fennel, Garlic and Mullein

Antispasmodics - Aniseed and Fennel

Demulcents - Licorice and Coltsfoot

Immune Boosters - Echinacea

Anti-Bacterial and Virals - Garlic and Echinacea

Out of the above I would choose Licorice, Echinacea, Garlic, Aniseed and Fennel. I would make the formula in this strength.

Formula
Licorice - 20%
Garlic - 15%
Echinacea - 15%

Aniseed - 30%
Fennel - 20%

Look these herbs up in the herbal and consider why I used them, there are three obvious ones for Licorice alone with the first being to force the assimilation of the formula into the body, second is its expectorant action and third is its demulcent action in case the throat is sore and raw. Next time you see a little kid eating heaps of licorice get them to open their mouth and look at their tongue which will be going black from the Licorice along with the throat etc and know that you are looking at the demulcent action of Licorice working by coating and soothing.

The most important reason that you use the Actions Method for Herbal Prescribing is so that you can concentrate the Actions which are most needed for example, if it's a Bacterial infection concentrate on the Anti Bacterials, if it's a Viral infection concentrate on the Anti Virals, hopefully you are now beginning to see the importance of working in actions for if you don't concentrate a large part of the battle on the causes you may have lost the battle from the start.

Read through all the Actions listed in Herbal Actions at the end of each body system in the book and then do a study in depth of at least five Actions of your choice making the first two the Anti Bacterials and Anti Virals. Start trying to train your mind into thinking in Actions.

How To Make Herbal Tinctures

Tinctures are made by steeping the Herb plant material in a mixture of alcohol and water. Alcohol is usually always used at a strength of 45%. The alcohol in this mixture will extract all the essential oils from the herb while the water will extract all that is water soluble, so between the both we are getting most of the medicinal properties out of the herb.

The proportions of herb to liquid are usually 1 part herb to 5 parts liquid. So find a suitable container (I use a big one liter preserving jar with a good sealing lid) and put into it 100grams of your chosen herb and to that add 500mls of our 45% solution of alcohol. Seal the lid and shake well for about a minute. Leave the jar on the window sill so the sun can shine on the jar for two weeks. The jar must be shaken for at least a minute every day.

After 2 weeks open and filter the contents of the jar. I use a large pouring jug into which I place a funnel and then place a coffee filter in the funnel and pour the jar contents through the funnel being careful not to let too much herb spill into the filter and block it up. When you get to the bottom of the jar you can crush the herb in your fist so as to extract the last of the liquid.

After this is completed you then get your chosen storage bottle, put a funnel into its neck followed by a coffee filter and then filter the jug into the bottle. Remember the solution should always be double filtered

Next we label the bottle, put the date, name and proportions eg 1 to 5 also state the recommended dose. Store in a cool and dark place. Most Professional Homoeopaths and Herbalists have access to pure alcohol so for them it is fairly easy to make tinctures while for the lay person they will probably have a hard time. A alternative is to use Vodka as strong as you can find it or find a way to twist the authorities arm into giving alcohol at 45%. Don't even try to get pure alcohol as it is dangerous and can turn people blind and they won't give it to you.

How To Make Infusions

Infusions are a bit like making a cup of tea except we don't use milk. Infusions are used for the soft parts of the herb such as the flowers, leaves and fine twigs. The proportions for infusions are 1 to 20 eg 1 part herb to 20 parts water. Infusions are used for the more water soluble herbs.

Infusions can be made from a single herb or from a combination of herbs and may be drunk hot or cold. The water should be just off the boil before being poured on the herb and if you are making a infusion of a herb strong in essential oils such as Peppermint always cover the top of the cup to stop the essential oils from escaping in steam while the infusion is brewing. Allow up to 10 minutes to brew. It is best to make herbal teas fresh each day. You can experiment on yourself by getting Chamomile and Peppermint tea bags from the supermarket. Use honey as a sweetener.

How To Make Decoctions

Decoctions are used for the more hard woody substances of the herb such as barks, berries or roots. The process of decoction is far more vigorous then infusion as it involves heating the plant material in cold water, bringing it to the boil and simmering for 20 to 40 minutes. The finished ratio for decoctions is again 1 part herb to 20 parts water, remember to add more water at the beginning so you wind up with the 1 to 20 after steam loss. This form of preparation is no good for the herbs that are high in essential oils as these will all be lost in the steam.

How To Make Poultices

Poultices are used to sooth, irritate or draw impurities from the skin so choose your required plants by the actions you need. A Poultice is used to apply a remedy to the skin with moist heat and slight pressure. To prepare a poultice bruise or crush the fresh medicinal parts of the herb you are using into a pulpy mass and add a little hot water if needed. If using dried herb moisten the material by mixing with a hot soft adhesive substance such as moist flower and cornmeal or as they did in the past a mixture of bread and milk. This can be done to the fresh herb if you want as well. For ease of application to the skin it is best to spread the mixture on cheese cloth and fold to the appropriate size or shape required. The cloth also helps by retaining the moisture and even allows you to tie it gently the affected area. Moisten the cloth with hot water periodically when and if needed. Hot water bottles can also be used to keep the poultice warm. Always keep some cloth between the skin when using irritant plants such as mustard and always wash the skin thoroughly after use.

Dosage For Forms Of Herbal Medicines

Herbs can be given to animals in several different forms depending on what best suites the herb, the ailment, and the condition of the animal and of what is available at the time and then most importantly the expense.

Herbal Extract - Are alcohol based and about the strongest herbal preparation you can get as they nearly extract everything from the herb. Generally the strength is every ml should be equivalent to one gram of the herb. Used and dosed the same as tinctures but the dose will always be less than what is used in a tincture. From this try to work out if the extra price is worth it. Supplier should give dosage.

Tincture - Is a weaker then Herbal Extracts but also made from alcohol. Dilute the appropriate number of drops in water for treatment. Supplier should give dosage.

Infusion - A infusion is like making a cup of tea out of the flowers and leaves and other soft parts of the herb. Add boiling water and cover so as all the essential oils don't escape in the steam and leave for 20 minutes.

Decoction - Usually made from the root, bark or seed and is simmered for a while to extract the medicinal properties. Usually dosed the same as infusions.

Powdered - These are usually made from roots and bark and given in doses from a teaspoon to tablespoon. These can also be infused and turned into a tea. Try to get powdered extracts as they are more the real thing instead of for example powdered Ginger at the supermarket.

Fresh Herb - This is the easiest way to medicate a horse just add a large handful of the leaves to the feed. Always check for woody parts and sharp stalks. For dangerous or strong herbs chop finely and mix thoroughly into moistened feed so no one animal eats too much.

Dried Herb - Most dried herb is usually cut, again run your hand through for wood or sharps. If you are growing the herb yourself cut up or grind and mix directly with the feed. Crushed herbs can also be mixed with water and formed into a pill for individual treatment or the whole stable can be dosed in a mix with feed.

Note - Always be guided by the recommended dose of the individual herb instead of working in generals.

Herbal General Animal Doses
Common Herbal Dosages for Herbivores
from Dr Hue Karreman

Form	*Goat*	*Cow*	*Horse*
Decoction	4oz	12oz	8oz
Extract Powder	1 tsp	2tbs	2tbs
Extract Tablet	3 to 5	10 to 15	10 to 15
Tincture	1 tsp	2 tbs	2 - 3 tbs

Herbivores require less per pound relative to the human or carnivoreDosage. These doses arc given two to three times daily.

Tbsp. = Tablespoon, roughly = to 15cc

Dr. Hubert Karreman is a 1995 graduate from the University of Pennsylvania School of Veterinary Medicine. He has been a dairy practitioner for 16 years in Lancaster, Pennsylvania. He is an internationally recognized expert in the non-antibiotic treatment of infectious disease.

Sheep - For sheep I would give a slightly smaller dose then that of the Goat as sheep are less hardy and have been severely genetically changed as I was trying to point out with my cover on the Sheep book.

Warning - Not all herbs in nature are of the same strength. For example if you gave the very strong herb Poke Root in tincture form at those doses the result would be a very sick animal, always remember herbs are not all the same. A safer way to go would be a comparison to the human dose to see if that is very low.

Notes

Calculating Correct Herbal Doses For Animals

Cats - 1/8 to 1/6 the dose for an adult human.

Dogs - Correspond to adult human dose according to weight.

Horse - 8 to 16 times the dose for an adult human.

Goats - 2 times the dose for an adult human.

Sheep - 1 1/2 times the dose for an adult human.

Cow - 12 to 24 times the dose for an adult human.

Swine - 1 to 3 times the dose for an adult human.

As mentioned in the warning above not all herbs are of the same strength so for this reason it is a good idea to always look at the human dose and if this dose seems to be lower than normal, if it is do your research into why. It might be a good idea to have a look at the herb Poke Root just to see what a strong herb looks like and can do.

Notes

Animal Herbal

Agrimony

Actions - Astringent, tonic, diuretic, vulnerary, cholagogue.

Used as a remedy for jaundice, it should be given to fasting animal as a drench or finely cut and mixed with bran, it is also a valuable astringent to stem bleeding and is a remedy for sore throats. Sprains are aided by a lotion made by boiling one handful of chopped Agrimony in one quart of brew made from wheaten bran. The combination of astringency and of bitter tonic properties make this a powerful herb for the digestive system. This is a good and gentle remedy for the young.

Uses - Diarrhea in the young, mucous colitis, spring tonic, indigestion, urinary incontinence and cystitis, as a gargle for sore throats and laryngitis and as a ointment or lotion for wounds and bruises.

Cautions - Not to be used during Pregnancy

Alfalfa

Rich in nitrates and vitamins is a good tonic food and a kidney cleanser. Excellent for all animals and poultry. Fodder, tonic, nervine, aids in healing allergies, arthritis, morning sickness, peptic ulcers, stomach ailments and bad breath, removes poisons from the body, neutralizes acids, is a excellent blood purifier and thinner, improves appetite and aids in the assimilation of protein, calcium and other nutrients.

Angelica

Actions - Expectorant, anti-spasmodic, diaphoretic, diuretic, carminative.

Useful expectorant for coughs, bronchitis and pleurisy especially when they are accompanied by fever, colds or influenza. The leaf can be used as a compress in inflammations of the chest. Its high oil content helps in intestinal colic and flatulence. Can ease rheumatic inflammations, in cystitis it acts as a urinary antiseptic.

Uses - Coughs, bronchitis, pleurisy, colic, wind, rheumatic inflammations, cystitis.

Aniseed

Actions - Expectorant, antispasmodic, carminative, parasiticide, aromatic.

Dogs like aniseed so much that it was once used as a bait by dog thieves. As a carminative it is unsurpassed. A important remedy for all digestive ailments including colic.

Uses - Gripping, intestinal colic, wind, as a expectorant in bronchitis, tracheitis, irritable coughing, whooping cough

External - The oil by itself will help in the control of lice and scabies..

Dose - Average dose for horses is one handful of seeds daily.

Arnica

Actions - Anti-inflammatory, vulnerary.

For external use only Homoeopathic preparations can be used internally. For the treatment of shock and pains from accidents, bruises, joint stiffness and wounds, swellings, paralysis, sprains, rheumatic conditions or where ever there is inflammation on the skin.

Caution - Do not apply to open wounds or broken skin.

Homoeopathy - Used from 3C to 200C orally for injury, bleeding, bruising, shock or for any conditions that feel bruised or have a bruised like feeling.

Astragalus

Actions - Immune-modulator, anti-viral, adaptogen, hypotensive, immune stimulant, adrenal tonic, diuretic, circulatory stimulant, vasodilator, blood tonic.

This herb should only be used in chronic diseases, as a preventative or in cases of fatigue especially in chronic diseases. Stimulates the natural production of interferon and intensifies the white cell destruction of germs.

A good tonic for strengthening the resistance to disease. Is very useful for animals in a state of chronic debility and fatigue by restoring the immune function. Use as a lung tonic to help expel toxins and pus in flu's, colds and sinusitis. Increases stamina and can accelerate wound healing, can help to replenish bone marrow. Strengthens the digestive system and aids adrenal gland function. This herb is used for cancer especially if the patient has had chemotherapy and helps aid them in their recovery.

Uses - Boosting immune system, disease preventative, fatigue, healing wounds. This is a good herb to use before and during a long distance or time consuming transportation.

Cautions - Should not be used in acute infections or fevers.

Barberry

Actions - Cholagogue, anti-emetic, bitter tonic, laxative, alterative, hypotensive, and antibacterial.

Good for correcting liver function and increasing the flow of bile. The herb is also a bitter tonic and mild laxative, use for weak and debilitated animals to strengthen and clean the system. Has been known to reduce enlarged spleens and also act against malaria. Its antibacterial properties have shown activity against strep, staff salmonella, shigella and eschorichia. This herb also dilates blood vessels thus lowering blood vessels.

Uses - Inflammation of the gallbladder, stones, liver problems, jaundice, arthritis, intestinal infections.

Cautions - Use only the dried plant and avoid during pregnancy.

Bear Berry - Uva Ursi

Actions - Diuretic, astringent, antiseptic and demulcent.

Bear Berry has a specific antiseptic and astringent effect on the membranes of the urinary system and will generally soothe tone and strengthen them. It is specifically used where there is gravel or ulceration in the kidneys or bladder. A very useful herb where there is cystitis.

Uses - Urinary infections, gravel and ulcerations in the urinary system also to soothe these areas.

Black Cohosh

Actions - Emmenagogue, anti-spasmodic, alterative, sedative.

Has hormone balancing properties, encourages oestrogen production, good for pets that loose hair after being spayed, painful or delayed menstruation, ovarian cramps, cramping pain, used to regain normal hormone activity, rheumatoid and osteoarthritis, muscular and neuralgic pains.

Blue Flag

Actions - Cholagogue, alterative, laxative, diuretic, anti-inflammatory.

Often called liver lily which shows its use in liver ailments. It acts as a general conditioner for the whole system and is also a gentle laxative. Stimulates the digestive glands. This is usually used with other blood cleansers and should be used in small doses at first in case it stirs up to much rubbish.

Uses - Treatment of all liver ailments, jaundice, gall bladder disorders, general tonic, appetizer, mild laxative, eczema, skin diseases, psoriasis.

Boswella

Actions - Anti-inflammatory, Antiarthritic, astringent

Good for use in any of the chronic inflammations in any body system.

Uses - Lung diseases especially of the chronic kind with inflammation, rheumatic diseases, diarrhea, dysentery, piles, STDs. It is also used in general weakness.

Broom

Actions - Cardioactive diuretic, hypertensive, peripheral vasoconstrictor, astringent.

Russian peasants use Broom tops as a very successful remedy for rabies. It is also used as a mild vermifuge. The flowers infused in hot milk (one handful to one pint) are used internally and externally to cure severe forms of skin ailments. The young twigs are mildly purgative.

Uses - Worms, skin ailments, rabies, dropsy, constipation, increases flow of urine in kidney ailments, used where there is a weak heart and low blood pressure, profuse menstruation.

Caution - Do not use in pregnancy and high blood pressure.

Burdock

Actions - Alterative, diuretic, bitter, antibacterial, anti-tumor.

It is used to treat conditions arising from an "overabundance" of toxins, such as boils, rashes and chronic skin problems. Helps to cleanse the body of waste products. Animals will not graze this herb with the exception of the ass, but the sliced and bruised roots are one of the finest blood cleansers known to herbalists. The bruised leaves applied externally are a remedy for ring worm and scabies. Soothing to the kidneys and a excellent diuretic. The juice is used internally for scabies and mites.

Uses - Remedy for all blood disorders, rheumatism, skin parasites , skin conditions resulting in dry scaly skin, psoriasis, eczema, dandruff, aids digestion and appetite, aids kidney function and helps with cystitis, speeds up the healing of wounds and ulcers. Use to reduce tumors.

Buchu

Actions - Diuretic, urinary antiseptic, digestive tonic, kidney tonic.

Used in any infection of the genito-urinary system such as cystitis, urethritis and prostatitis. Especially useful in painful and burning urination. Good kidney tonic. Used to treat blood in the urine, stones and chronic urinary infections especially if started by colon bacteria.

Cayenne

Actions - Stimulant, carminative, tonic, sialagogue, rubefacient, anti-septic.

Used as a catalyst to help push herbal formulas into the body. Aids heart failure (a few drops on the side of the mouth), stimulates the heart, helps heal ulcers of the stomach and colon, cayenne powder sprinkled on a open wound stops bleeding, flatulent dyspepsia, colic. Externally it is used as a rubefacient in problems like lumbago and rheumatic pains.

Caution - High doses on an empty stomach can cause gut irritation and eventually ulcers

Calendula

Actions - Anti-inflammatory, astringent, vulnerary, anti-fungal, cholagogue, emmenagogue.

Goats and sheep seek it out, the flowers are tonic and a good heart medicine they possess restorative powers over the arteries and veins, the flowers are also fed to make miserable fretting animals cheerful, also used for liver problems, vomiting, internal ulcers.

Uses - Cuts, grazes, infected sores, fungal infections, any skin inflammations, regulates the oil production of the skin so is good for acne, to stop bleeding, bruises and sprains, skin ulcers and minor burns and scolds, healing, soothing, anti-microbial. Use as a lotion to clean wounds, one of our main germicides for wounds and if Hypericum is added to the lotion you may prevent tetanus as well.

Use externally as a lotion (1 to 20) or a cream.

Caution - Calendula closes wounds rapidly so make sure they are very clean and no foreign bodies remain.

Cat Mint

Actions - Carminative, antispasmodic, diaphoretic, sedative, astringent.

This herb is also known as Catnip. Cats and other creatures eat this plant and also give themselves a massage in it. This plant sometimes causes cats to grow pensive and dreamy. This is a old traditional cold and flu remedy especially ones with fever. Has a action on the digestive system easing stomach upsets, dyspepsia, wind and colic. Used for diarrhea of the young. Good for nervous, stressed or restless animals.

Cats Claw

Actions - Anti oxidant, immune stimulant, anti-inflammatory, anti-fungal, anti-rheumatic, anti-viral, anti-tumor, anti-microbial.

To alleviate allergic sinus type conditions, boost the immune system, asthma, bursitis, Candida, immune deficiency disorders, chronic inflammatory diseases, auto immune conditions.

Cautions - Dont use during pregnancy.

Celery Seed

Actions - Anti rheumatic, diuretic, carminative, sedative, alterative, hypotensive.

The main use for this herb is in the treatment of rheumatism, arthritis and gout. Celery seed can help soothe the nerves and relieve pain and also aids the body in the removal of uric acid. A good cleansing, mildly diuretic herb, useful in ridding the system of an accumulation of waste products. An improvement in circulation of fluids encourages a horse to drink and sweat more easily. Celery seed mixed with food aids in the digestion of protein. A very good digestive tonic if the horse is run down with little appetite.

Uses - Arthritis, hyperacidity, pain, hypertension, digestion, urinary tract infections

Centaury

Actions - Bitter, aromatic, mild nervine, gastric stimulant, chologogue, febrifuge, vermafuge.

Use whenever a gastric stimulant is required especially in cases of anorexia and liver weakness. This is a good herb for use in the young.

Uses - For digestive ailments, jaundice, as a vermafuge including liver fluke, use externally for lice, wounds and warts. In the past it was also used as a birth remedy.

Chamomile

Actions - Carminative, sedative, anti-spasmodic, anti-inflammatory, analgesic and anti-septic.

It is a famed blood cleanser and pain reducer, reduces tumors (poultice), remedy for female ailments, inflamed gums, use for blood and skin disorders, aches and pains, external and internal inflammations, delayed menstruation, acid uterus and all female ailments, cleanser and toner of the digestive tract, it is well documented as having anti-inflammatory activity and is also beneficial in reducing allergic responses as it contains a number of anti-histamine chemicals. In addition, it is recognized as being ulcer-protective through its healing effect on the mucosa of the gastro-intestinal tract, expels worms and parasites, improves and helps appetite. Good for nervous and hyperactive horses as it calms them without making them tired.

Uses - Indigestion, colic, diarrhea, teething, anxiety, insomnia, nervous upsets, slowing down hyperactive horses, flatulence. Good all round tonic for the nervous system especially for nervous animals.

Chaparral

Actions - Alterative, astringent, diuretic, tonic, powerful antioxidant, anti-arthritic, anti-rheumatic, anti-cancer, anti-tumor, dissolves calculi, anti-biotic.

Uses - Used in kidney problems and stones and for rheumatism and arthritis. Aids in healing skin blemishes, acne, allergies, promotes hair growth, acts as a natural anti biotic, cataracts, has a action on cancer.

Chaste Tree

Actions - Emmenagogue, galactagogue, Tonic for the reproductive organs.

More of a hormone balancer by working directly on the pituitary gland though is more of a normalizing herb, usually increases the progesterone levels therefore increasing the chance of pregnancy. Supporting the progesterone level is extremely helpful in counteracting the irritability and unpredictability that can happen with mares in season making them more comfortable, cooperative and safer to handle. Though this herb is primarily used to balance hormonal irregularities in mares it can also be used to inhibit the sex hormones of stallions if their behavior is thought dangerous or seen to be causing them a loss in condition. Useful on its own or in combination with herbs specific for hormonal balance.

Used for endometriosis, fibroids, infertility and threatened miscarriages.

Chickweed

Actions - Healing, anti-inflammatory, astringent, emollient.

Rich in copper, highly tonic food for the digestive system and a remedy for all stomach ailments, allergies, colon problems, constipation, piles, rheumatism, skin problems, eczema, psoriasis, itching, irritation, cuts and wounds.

Uses - One of the main uses of this herb is for itching skin conditions whether from insect bites or eczema like conditions. Has wound healing and demulcent properties.

Cleavers

Actions - Alterative, diuretic, anti-inflammatory, astringent, tonic, anti-cancer.

A lymphatic tonic with alterative and diuretic actions which can be used in a wide range of problems where the lymphatic system is involved. The plant is very rich in minerals and silica, gives good strong texture to the hair of animals and strengthens the hoofs. Also used to ease swollen legs and joints, support the lymphatic and endocrine systems and encourage the elimination of toxins, is also helpful if your horse experiences muscle tightening during or after exercise. All animals eat it and poultry especially seek it hence its popular name of goose grass. Good for skin ailments.

Uses - Tonic, eczema, abscesses and tumors, cancerous growths, swollen glands, tonsillitis, psoriasis, cystitis.

Coltsfoot

Actions - Expectorant, anti tussive, demulcent, anti-catarrhal, diuretic.

The Latin name means banish cough.. Coltsfoot combines a soothing expectorant action with a anti spasmodic action. There are useful zinc levels in this plant. Consider this herb in any respiratory problem.

Uses - Coughs, pneumonia, asthma, pleurisy, TB, sedative powers in epilepsy, chronic or acute bronchitis, emphysema, cystitis.

Externally - A poultice is used for abscess, ulcers, boils, earache and toothache.

Comfrey

Actions - Demulcent, astringent, healing, expectorant.

Once widely cultivated as a fodder plant, sheep and cows eat it greedily, the impressive wound healing powers of comfrey are partially due to allantoin which stimulates cell proliferation and speeds the healing process inside and out. Has been used for thousands of years as a herb with abilities to mend broken bones. Has the same result on wounds, tendons, fractures, sprains, ulcers and cartilage.

Uses - Its old name is knit bone and that describes well what it does. Comfrey also guards against scar tissue from developing incorrectly, all internal hemorrhages including uterine, reunion of wound and fractures, internal ulcers, ruptures, pulmonary problems, bronchitis, irritable cough, ulcerative colitis, skin ulcers and varicose veins.

Corn Silk

Actions - Diuretic, demulcent, tonic, antiseptic, antilithic.

A soothing diuretic that is helpful in any irritation of the membranes of the urinary system. Combined with other herbs in the treatment of cystitis, urethritis and prostatitis. Cleanses and soothes the urinary system.

Cranesbill

Action - Strong astringent, anti-inflammatory, vulnerary.

One of the best astringents known for internal and external use and is palatable to most animals.

Uses - Dysentery and diarrhea especially in the old and young, piles, duodenal or gastric ulcers, uterine hemorrhage or any internal bleeding especially of the digestive and respiratory systems, douche in leucorrhoea, treatment of wounds.

Cranberry

Actions - Urinary antiseptic

Cranberry inhibits the adhesion of bacteria to the urinary pipe lines so each time water is passed the bacteria is flushed out thus preventing recolonization.

Dandelion

Actions - Diuretic, cholagogue, anti-rheumatic, laxative, tonic

The leaves of the Dandelion plant are generally fed to horses during spring as the herb assists with cleansing the blood. They are high in iron and calcium as well as Vitamins A, B, and D and are traditionally used as a tonic to stimulate the bladder.

The herb is blood cleansing and tonic, it has a important effect on the hepatic system and is a supreme jaundice curative herb, the leaves strengthen the enamel of the teeth and the white   juices of the freshly crushed stem dissolves warts, the plant is well grazed by goats, horses will take quantities of the leaves when cut and well mixed with bran. Dandelion Root is helpful for horses recovering from an illness or a reaction to vaccination. Being a tonic, this herb assists to clean the liver, kidneys and blood and is high in potassium and magnesium. Excellent for anemia because it is high in iron, calcium, copper and vitamins, useful in kidney and bladder problems, skin eruptions, sluggish blood flow, weak arteries, all liver complaints, jaundice, constipation, gallbladder problems and rheumatism.

Devils Claw

Actions - Anti-inflammatory, pain killer, hepatic, anti-rheumatic, alterative.

Used for its analgesic and anti-inflammatory properties, it is useful for treating pain in a range of joint and muscular problems. The bitter action of Devils Claw stimulates and tones the digestive system. Good for reducing inflammation in arthritis, gout and rheumatism. Aids the body in the elimination of uric acid. This plant also aids liver and gallbladder complaints.

Caution- Use with demulcent herbs to save irritating the tummy, don't use on horses with ulcers.

Dong Quai

Actions - Emmenagogue, antispasmodic, analgesic, uterine tonic ,vasodilator, hormone balancer, alterative.

Known regulator for the female reproductive system. Some of its compounds stimulate the uterus while others relax the uterus. The compounds that stimulate the uterus are water soluble and are absorbed into the body from teas and capsules. The compounds that relax the uterus are soluble in alcohol and are provided by tinctures. This herb may stop cramping, and ease the pain of ovarian cysts. The Chinese use this herb for abnormal menstruation, suppressed flow, painful or difficult menstruation. This herb is also good for the treatment of psoriasis. Dong Quai also helps with , asthma, bronchitis, emphysema and improves the function of the lungs. Builds and improves circulation as well as disperses congestion in the pelvic area.

Cautions - Avoid during pregnancy and in cases with diarrhea and dysentery.

Echinacea

Actions - Immune stimulant, anti-microbial, anti-inflammatory, alterative, healing.

Is a infection fighter active against strep bacteria (abscesses and boils), a blood cleanser, (blood poisons, snake bites, poisonous insects) and a glandular and lymphatic system cleanser. Use it particularly for respiration infections and for any disease above the waist. This is one of our main immune boosters for the acute diseases. Use as a prophylactic to protect horses from infections especially when traveling.

Uses - All infections, depressed immune function, inflammatory conditions, allergies, effective against both bacteria and viruses.

Warning - Do not use continually as you will burn out the immune system give a few weeks break after 3 weeks. Beware also in the use of allergies for you could be building up the immune system just to attack itself.

Elecampane

Actions - Expectorant, antitussive, anti-bacterial, antifungal, diaphoretic, stomachic, demulcent.

This herb is meant to be named after Helen of Troy and is a very ancient herb used for thousands of years especially by the Romans. Specific for irritating bronchial coughs, lots of catarrh, has a soothing and anti-bacterial action.

Mainly used for treating chronic coughs, bronchitis and asthma especially in the young. . It is also used for digestive problems. Elecampane also contains Alantolactone which helps to expel intestinal parasites such as pin worm. A external wash can help deter Scabies.

Uses - Bronchitis, emphysema, asthma and digestive problems. In the past was used for TB.

Elder

Actions - Diaphoretic, diuretic, anti-catarrhal, expectorant.

Most animals will graze on elder. Used for the treatment of all gastric, hepatic, and pulmonary ailments, all fevers, skin disorders especially scabies and ring worm, externally as a insecticide.

Leaves - Externally emollient and vulnerary (bruises, sprains and wounds). Internally used as a purgative, expectorant, diuretic and Diaphoretic. Topically the lotion makes a anti-inflammatory wash, salve, eyewash and gargle for sore throats.

Flowers - Diaphoretic and Anti catarrhal. Use for colds and flu.

Berries - Diaphoretic and Anti catarrhal. The uses are similar to the flowers but the berries are used for rheumatism. The berries have been used as a nutrient rich tonic given after birth to help build the blood.

Eye Bright

Actions - Anti-inflammatory, astringent, anti-catarrhal.

As the name says this is one of the main herbs in the treatment of eye problems. The aerial (above ground) parts of the plant are used. As its name suggests, it helps eye problems by relieving inflammation and tightening mucous membranes and is specifically used in treating conjunctivitis and blepharitis. Used for infections and allergic conditions affecting the eyes, middle ear, sinuses and nasal passages.

The plant is also nervine, tonic and astringent. Its use is both internal and external strengthening greatly the eyes nerves when used so. The high potassium and sulphur content of the plant make it also of value in treatment of gastric ailments especially insufficiency of gastric juices. Acts as a internal medicine for the constitutional tendency to eye weakness.

Uses- Best known for its use in the eye where it is helpful in acute or chronic inflammations, stinging and weeping eyes, over sensitivity to light, conjunctivitis, allergies, sinusitis, ulcers and general eye weakness.

Fennel

Actions - Carminative, aromatic, anti-spasmodic, stimulant, galactagogue, expectorant.

The herb possesses highly antiseptic and tonic properties. The primary use of fennel is to relieve bloating, but it also settles stomach pain, stimulates the appetite and is diuretic and anti-inflammatory. Peasants drive their flocks to feed upon it owing to the abundance of milk that the herb produces and the sweet odor that it imparts upon the milk. (if the animal is not native they can over gorge and poison themselves).

Arabs use fennel poultices to resolve old and hard tumors.

Uses - Gastric ailments, relieves flatulence and colic, stimulates appetite, inflammation of the bowels, acute constipation (raw roots daily), fevers, cramps, worms, indigestion, all eye ailments, bronchitis, coughs, muscular and rheumatic pains use the oil. Externally used as a eye wash to treat eye infections.

Fenugreek

Actions - Expectorant, demulcent, tonic, carminative, galactagogue, alterative, restorative.

Strongly aromatic herb, and the seeds of the plant are used. It contains a volatile oil, flavonoids, mucilage, protein, Vitamins A, B & C, alkaloids, saponins and some minerals. The seeds can aid in recovery from illness and to encourage weight gain. This is a herb well worth getting to know not just because of its tonic properties but for its rubbish removing actions especially in mucous thick chronic diseases such as sinusitis. Always use cleansing herbs like this one slowly and at a low doses especially when using for long periods of time. The plant possesses highly aromatic seeds having a powerful disinfectant, emollient and lubricant properties. The feeding value of these is about equal to linseed. It is one of the great fattening herbs. The perfect sister herb for garlic enhancing all its powers. Very tonic and eagerly sought by all animals. Rich in vitamins and nitrates, calcium and phosphorus. The whole plant is used.

Uses - Treatment for all gastric weaknesses and ailments, nerves and neuralgia, female ailments including failing milk supply, allergies, bronchitis, anemia, bruises, colitis, coughs, diabetes, fever, flu, hay fever, headache, migraines, lung problems, sinus congestion, ulcers, reduces inflammation, has a reputation for stimulating and developing breasts.

Externally - It can be used as a poultice for relief of abscess, boils, tumors and running sores.

Caution - Avoid during pregnancy as it can be a uterine stimulant.

Feverfew

Actions - Anti-inflammatory, vasodilator, relaxant, digestive bitter, uterine stimulant.

It is one of the most important aids for female ailments the plant exerting remarkable powers over the uterus, the whole plant is used. Has a good reputation for migraine headaches, may help with arthritis when it is in the inflammatory stage, painful periods. Feverfew inhibits the manufacture of substances causing inflammation.

Uses - Digestive aid and tonic, treatment for all female irregularities especially scanty or failing menses, inflamed or weak uterus and uterine and vaginal ulcers, abortion, difficult labor, retained afterbirth, arthritis, inflammations.

Cautions - Do not use during pregnancy because of the stimulant action on the womb. The fresh leaves may cause mouth ulcers in sensitive people.

Figwort

Actions - Alterative, diuretic, mild purgative, heart stimulant.

Used for any skin condition where there is itching and irritation. This herb cleans out the system especially the blood and bowels. Can be used has a heart stimulant or for poor circulation but is contraindicated for this when there is a rapid heartbeat (tachycardia)

Uses - Failing or weak heart, eczema, psoriasis, acne, cradle cap, mild laxative. Externally use for boils, burns ,eczema, rashes, ringworm and wounds.

Fumitory

Actions - Diuretic, cholagogue, laxative, alterative.

Has a long history of use in the treatment of skin problems such as eczema and acne, its action is probably due to a general cleansing mediated via the kidneys and liver. Cows and sheep seek it out greedily. The whole plant is used.

Uses - All forms of liver ailments and gallbladder problems, skin eruptions, eczema, wounds, scabies, ulcerated mouth, inflamed liver, jaundice, biliousness.

Garlic

Actions - Immune stimulant, anti-bacterial, anti-viral, anti-fungal, anti-septic, anti-oxidant, diaphoretic, cholagogue, hypotensive, anti-spasmodic, vermifuge and many more.

The plant is rich in volatile oil and sulphur and because of its remarkable penetrating, disinfecting and mucous expelling powers garlic is a valuable basic remedy for the treatment of all ailments in which the cleansing of the blood stream and expulsion of mucous accumulations is required. Garlic can be used to prevent and treat respiratory infections. Anyone who has had garlic breath has experienced this herb's aromatic compounds being excreted through their lungs which is why garlic's active ingredients can be so effective for respiratory complaints. Garlic is extremely effective in dissolving and cleansing cholesterol from the blood stream, it stimulates the digestive tract, kills worms, parasites and harmful bacteria, normalizes blood pressure, reduces fever, gas and cramps.

Uses- All infections, coughs, colds, flu, bronchitis, all fevers, pulmonary conditions, gastric and skin complaints, rheumatism, all worms and also liver fluke, mange, ringworm, ticks and lice.

Acts on Bacteria, Viruses and Internal Parasites.

Externally - You can use garlic for ring worm and ear ache, to disinfect wounds and sores, parasitical infections.

Guaiacum

Actions - Anti rheumatic, anti-inflammatory, laxative, diaphoretic, diuretic, alterative, peripheral circulatory stimulant.

Specific for rheumatic complaints with lots of inflammation, aids in the treatment of gout and can be used here as a preventative. Care must be taken with this herb especially in allergic conditions.

Gentian

Actions - Bitter, gastric stimulant, sialagogue, cholagogue.

The root is the medicinal part. Gentian is one of the most important tonic herbs being considered the Prince of the Bitters. Quells vomiting when all other herbs fail, promotes the production of saliva, gastric juices and bile along with stimulating peristalsis, indicated where there is a lack of appetite and sluggishness of the digestive system.

Uses - Treatment of all forms of digestive weakness, vomiting, nervous ailments including hysteria, malaria, to improve the appetite of all poor feeders.

Ginger

Actions- Carminative, anti-inflammatory,

vasodilator, circulatory stimulant, diaphoretic, anti-emetic.

The therapeutic benefits of ginger are largely due to its volatile oil and oleoresin content. Ginger is an excellent remedy for many digestive complaints, including nausea, colic, wind and indigestion. Its antiseptic properties also make it beneficial for gastro-intestinal infections. For the older, arthritic horse, ginger is a useful maintenance herb. It stimulates the circulatory system and helps blood flow and increases stamina. Aids in fighting colds, colitis, digestive disorders, wind, increases saliva.

Uses- Indigestion, nausea, feverish conditions especially when chills are present, travel sickness especially sea sickness, dyspepsia, colic, flatulence.

Caution - Don't use large doses on a empty stomach..

Ginkgo Biloba

Actions - Anti fungal, anti-bacterial, antioxidant, anti tussive, astringent, expectorant, anti-allergy and anti-inflammatory but mainly used for its Peripheral Vaso - Dilator effects.

Is native to Northern China and is considered the world's oldest tree species. This herb can be helpful for a horse resuming work after a spell, or for older horses that are sound for riding but are slowing down. Due to its effect on peripheral and cerebral (brain) circulation it can assist the blood supply to limbs, and general alertness. (think of mixing with

Hawthorn). The leading symptoms pointing to Ginkgo are cold hands and feet. This herb opens up the femoral arteries and neck arteries increasing blood supply to those areas thus improving the function of everything in those areas by the increase in oxygen and blood sugar. For the old animal thinking and seeing may improve and walking may also become a bit easier. In asthma ginkgo helps reduce the inflammation response making the attacks less severe. The herb is safe to use as a tonic. This is a good herb to take in a mixed antioxidant formula.

Ginseng (Panax)

Actions - Anti depressive, restorative, tonic, adaptogen, stimulating adrenal agent, increases resistance and improves mental and physical performance.

This is the strong ginseng, think twice about giving it to a horse with a shy and sensitive nature its more for the outgoing and competitive nature. This herb can help with depression especially when caused by debility and exhaustion. It can be used in general for exhaustion and weakness. Used to increase mental and physical performance, to improve concentration, vigilance and work efficiency, stamina, for combating internal or external stress factors of any kind - athletics, endurance activities, aging, surgery, disease, infections, cold, but especially degenerative conditions and problems of old age. This is a good herb for infertility.

Cautions - Avoid with high blood pressure, during acute infections. This herb can be over stimulating for some. Use month on month off.

Ginseng Siberian

Actions - Adaptogen, vaso dilator, increases stamina, circulatory stimulant.

This herb is very similar to the one above but is a milder version and can be used all the time as it does not build up in the system like Panax Ginseng. Always consider giving a break from herbs as it is not good to use any herb all the time except maybe Hawthorn for a failing heart.

Goldenrod

Actions - Ant catarrhal, anti-inflammatory, antiseptic, diaphoretic, carminative, diuretic, astringent, tonic, hypotensive.

It is famed as a wound herb, is a important remedy for female disorders, all cattle eat it and it brings them into good appetite and gives bloom, the whole plant is used, traditionally used for inflammation, upper respiratory catarrh, use with other herbs for influenza, flatulent dyspepsia, as a urinary anti-inflammatory and anti-septic, cystitis, urethritis and also used for urinary stones. This herb is also used for arthritis.

Uses - A powerful digestive aid, treatment of jaundice, kidney problems.

Externally - For wounds, to stop bleeding, cleansing gangrenous conditions.

Gravel Root

Actions - Diuretic, anti-lithic, anti-rheumatic.

Used primarily for kidney stones and gravel. In urinary infections such as cystitis and urethritis it may be used with benefit, good in the systemic treatment of rheumatism and gout.

Grindelia

Actions - Antispasmodic, expectorant, hypotensive, cardiac relaxant, diuretic, tonic.

This plant comes from the Americas and has long been used for asthma, it acts to relax the smooth muscles and is good for asthma and bronchitis especially when these are associated with a rapid heartbeat and a nervous disposition. Also used for whooping cough and respiratory catarrh. Ellingwood a famous Herbalist from the past considered it a specific for asthmatic breathing. Because of the relaxing effect on the heart and pulse there may be a lowering of blood pressure. Has a tonic effect on the lungs and kidneys and is mildly diuretic.

Topically this herb has been used for eczema, insect bites, poison ivy and burns.

Caution - Don't use for those with weak hearts or low blood pressure.

Hawthorn

Actions - Cardiac tonic, hypotensive, adaptogen. Strengthens the muscles and nerves of the heart, aids in relieving emotional stress, regulates high and low blood pressure, helps combat arteriosclerosis and heart disease. With regard to horses, hawthorn's effects on peripheral circulation makes it valuable for treating conditions such as navicular and laminitis. Indeed, horses and ponies suffering from these ailments have been observed seeking out the new growth on hawthorn bushes. This is more of a balancing herb, if the blood pressure is high or low the herb will balance it if the electrical activity is playing up with rapid or erratic heart beat it will try to balance it. Strengthens and helps to remove plaques from the blood vessels. This is a herb for taking in the long term.

Uses - As a tonic to the circulatory system and to strengthen the heart.

Hops

Actions - Sedative, hypnotic, antiseptic, astringent, nervine, bitter digestive tonic, antibacterial. Famed for its tonic and nervine properties, pain reliever, sleep inducer, anti-septic, vermifuge, tension that leads to restlessness, headache, indigestion, mucous colitis. Good for when digestive problems are caused by worry or nerves. Good for nervous horses. One of the main remedies for IBS. Acts on the central nervous system and calms and eases anxiety. Hops contains estrogenic substances which could interfere with hormone therapy.

Uses - Treatment of all digestive ailments, general debility, failing appetite, wasting, fevers, eczema, worms, to quietens restless animals.

Externally - Eczema.

Horehound (White)

Actions - Expectorant, anti-spasmodic, bitter, digestive, vulnerary.

Is one of the most important pectoral herbs a famed cough and throat remedy, the bitter action stimulates the flow of bile and thus improves digestion.

Uses - Treatment of cough, pneumonia, pleurisy, bronchitis, TB, atrophy of the lungs, ear disorders, canker, diarrhea, inflammation of the liver, jaundice.

Horse Chestnut

Actions - Circulatory tonic, astringent, anti-inflammatory, nutritive.

Has a action on the vessels of the circulatory system especially veins where it seems to increase their strength and tone. Can be used internally and externally on the veins themselves. The nuts in the past were fed to animals as a tonic food and was also said to enrich the milk. It also was used in the past to treat the cough of horses and this is where it gets its name.

Uses - Inflammation of veins, varicose veins, piles, capillary weakness

Cautions - Avoid with kidney disease.

Horseradish

Actions - Stimulant, carminative, mild laxative, diuretic, antiseptic, tonic.

It's hot properties make it valuable in expelling worms, stimulating appetite and as a general tonic, it is a internal antiseptic, helps to remove excess urine from the system and stones from the bladder, urinary infection, all parts of the plant are used, can be used in influenza and fevers, eases wind and gripping pains in the digestive system, bronchitis.

Uses - Worm and kidney treatment, to reduce tumors, asthma, bronchitis, sinusitis, remedy for lack of appetite and over thinness.

Externally - As a poultice for swellings.

Horsetail

Actions - Astringent, diuretic, vulnerary.

Goats eat the plant but it is not a good food for cows, excellent astringent for the genito-urinary system reducing bleeding and healing wounds thanks to its high silica content, inflammation of the prostrate, tones and astringes the urinary system making it a good remedy for incontinence and bed wetting. Use for kidney stones as the high silica content erodes stones. May speed up the healing of bone, flesh and cartilage due to its high mineral content.

Uses - Nasal hemorrhage, laryngitis, intestinal ulcer, inflammation of the uterus, vagina and bladder, dysentery, enlarged anal glands, obesity, dropsy, a strong dose dissolves stones in the bladder.

Caution - If used over a long period it may decrease vitamin B1.

Hypericum (St Johns Wort)

Actions - Anti-inflammatory, astringent, anti-viral, anti-spasmodic, nervine, vulnerary, antibacterial.

The name St Johns Wort came from the Knights of St John of Jerusalem who used the herb to treat battle wounds.

Uses - Taken internally has a sedative and pain reducing effect, neuralgic pain, anxiety, tension, rheumatic pain, sciatica, for pains that shoot along the nerves, as a lotion it will speed the healing of wounds and bruises and is used where there is damage to the nerve rich areas, varicose veins and mild burns. Good for inflamed joints and rheumatic pain. In humans recently the herb has become popular to use as a antidepressant especially for cases of anxiety. Use as a lotion on wounds especially in the nerve rich areas such as the lips and fingers. As a lotion it is commonly mixed with Calendula, Homoeopaths call this lotion Hypercal.

Caution - Animals that overdose on Hypericum become photosensitive and have to be locked in the barn for a while so as not to become sun burnt.

Hyssop

Actions - Anti spasmodic, expectorant, antiviral, nervine, diaphoretic, sedative, carminative.

A important plant in pectoral complaints because it removes mucous accumulations and also tones up the membranes and fortifies the whole system along with being a respiratory antiviral. Is a mild vermifuge the Nordic countries use it as a vermifuge for delicate lambs and kids. Coughs, bronchitis, chronic catarrh, colds and flu's, anxiety states, hysteria, petit mal.

Uses - Treatment of cough especially the more spasmodic coughs such as whooping, sore throat, pneumonia, pleurisy, TB, or any respiratory disease, worms, eye disorders, conjunctivitis.

Juniper

Actions - Diuretic, antiseptic, carminative, anti-rheumatic.

The whole plant is a tonic and nerve stimulant, excellent anti septic in conditions like cystitis, stimulating to the kidney nephrons (avoid in kidney disease), the bitter action aids digestion and eases flatulent colic.

Uses - Treatment of inflamed liver and kidneys, gallstones, jaundice, obesity, sciatica, rheumatism, blood ailments, acid milk, malaria.

Caution - Avoid in kidney disease. Avoid in

pregnancy.

Kelp

Actions - Antihypothyroid, anti-rheumatic, nutritive,
Used mainly for under active thyroid (iodine) especially when it is thought to be the cause of overweight. Helps in the relief of rheumatism internally and externally. Added to feed for nutrition. Can be used to slim fat horses. Make sure that iodine isn't in any of the supplements you are already giving. It is good for coat and hoof conditions.

Ladys Mantle

Actions - Astringent, diuretic, anti-inflammatory, emmenagogue, vulnerary.
This herb has a affinity to the womb where it helps with pain, bleeding and getting the cycle back to normal. Horses, goats and sheep seek out the herb, the plant is tonic and an important fortifier for the blood and walls of the arteries, it is a old herbal remedy for diabetes, reduces period pains and excessive bleeding, diarrhea, sores, ulcers a good menopause herb.

Uses - Treatment for lack of appetite, wasting, weak blood, sluggish blood, all weaknesses of the arteries, heart disease, taken from one period to another it is reputed to aid conception in barren animals.

Lemon Balm (Melissa)

Actions - Carminative, antispasmodic, anti-depressive, diaphoretic, hypotensive, emmenagogue, nervine, rejuvenating tonic, Anti-viral.

In the past this plant was used to attract bees by rubbing it all around a new hive and the smell made the bees want to stay. The name Melissa is Greek for honey bee. The Arabs say it gives intelligence to any animal that feeds upon it.

Relieves spasms in the digestive tract and is used in flatulent dyspepsia. Good for digestive problems brought on from worry, anxiety and stress. Has a tonic effect on the heart and circulatory system causing mild vasodilatation of the peripheral blood vessels which can help to lower blood pressure and also may calm the electrical activity of the heart. Has also been used in animals for retained afterbirth and as a anti-viral for infections such as herpes.

Caution - Can sometimes lower thyroid function.

Licorice

Actions - Expectorant, demulcent, anti-inflammatory, adrenal agent, anti-spasmodic, mild laxative.

The root part is used , possessing unique pectoral and emollient properties, it is also nutritive and slightly laxative, It contains the building blocks of hormones, has a marked effect on the endocrine system, catarrh, gastric and peptic ulcers, abdominal colic. Its ability to soothe irritated mucous membranes and to break up phlegm and ease coughing sees licorice employed in respiratory conditions, coughing, bronchitis, and chest colds. Can be used for treating inflammatory and allergic conditions.. Licorice has effects on the adrenal glands which are protective, restorative, tonic and stimulatory. These properties can aid the horse which is recovering from steroid therapy or abuse.

Uses - Treatment of cough, inflamed throat, pneumonia, pleurisy, TB, all catarrhal conditions, gallstones, chronic constipation, mild worms in young animals, female infertility, pains of colic.

Caution - Do not use with high blood pressure. Long term use depletes potassium which raises the blood pressure. Don't use with steroids.

Lime Blossom (Linden)

Actions - Nervine, antispasmodic, diaphoretic, diuretic, mild astringent.

Possesses powerful nervine and blood cleansing properties, used for fits and nervous twitching of all kinds including epilepsy, a good tonic for bees, nervous tension, as a prophylactic against arteriosclerosis, migraines, feverish colds and flu.

Uses - Treatment of all nervous ailments especially epilepsy, twitching, vertigo, good for colds and to remove the slime and mucous from the system, treatment of vomiting, heart pains, fevers, treatment of tumors by poultice.

Marsh Mallow

Actions - Demulcent, anti-inflammatory, expectorant, astringent.

Its therapeutic effects are largely due to its significant mucilage and pectin content, aided by its anti-inflammatory properties. The foliage of the mallow is eaten by all animals, the roots are the main part used for internal medicine and also the leaves which are especially used for inflammation of the stomach and bowel and especially used for ulcers, it contains over half its weight in sweet tasting mucilage which possess unique properties of lubricating, soothing and healing. A poultice can be used for all inflammatory conditions. Horses who have colic, or who are scouring, can benefit from the soothing and healing effects of marshmallow also see Slippery Elm. Consider using as a supplement for horses prone to colic and ulcers. Marshmallow can also be used to soothe inflamed and irritated mucous membranes of the respiratory and urinary systems. Dry coughs, sore throats, urinary tract inflammation and cystitis have all been relieved by the effects of marshmallow.

Uses - Treatment of sore throats, pulmonary catarrhs, pleurisy, cystitis, diarrhea, dysentery, ulcers, bowel inflammations and hemorrhages.

Externally - All skin eruptions, abrasions, swellings, inflammations, bruises, sore inflamed udders.

Marigold see Calendula

Meadowsweet

Actions - Anti-inflammatory, anti-rheumatic, antacid, anti-emetic, stomachic, astringent.

A important fever and diarrhea herb, the gypsies use as a spring tonic for their animals, eaten plentifully by goats and sheep, acts to protect and soothe the mucous membranes of the digestive tract reducing excess acidity and easing nausea, heart burn, hyperacidity, gastritis, peptic ulcers. This herb is a good acid balancer and is good for correcting over acid systems. Meadowsweet is the forerunner of aspirin as this is the first herb it was synthesized from in 1835 but as this herb contains its own buffering agents it is gentle on the stomach. Used to help reduce inflammation and for pain relief in case of arthritic conditions. Useful alone or in combination with other herbs for effective pain management.

Uses - Fevers, arthritis, diarrhea and the above mentioned.

Caution - Avoid if sensitive to salicylates.

Mistletoe

Actions - Nervine, hypotensive, cardiac depressant, possibly anti tumour.

It will quiet soothe and tone the nervous system, acts directly on the vagus nerve to reduce heart rate while strengthening the walls of the peripheral capillaries, reduces blood pressure and eases arteriosclerosis, nervous tachycardia, headache due to high blood pressure.

Uses - Treatment of nervous ailments, epilepsy, hysteria, heart tonic, uterine and vaginal bleeding.

Milk Thistle - St Mary's Thistle

Actions - Cholagogue, galactagogue, demulcent.

This herb is said to rejuvenate the liver, for problems like hepatitis it is used alone at first as it drains the liver probably by its action of stimulating the gallbladder to release bile. Much of the therapeutic benefit of the seeds is attributed to a group of potent antioxidant bioflavonoids, known together as silymarin, which are able to guard and stabilize cell membranes, preventing the invasion of toxins, as well as enhance the regeneration of liver cells already damaged by detoxification processes. for horses who have suffered liver damage from poisons, infections, high worm burdens, reactions to worming drugs, or excessive drug use. Can be taken long term and needs be taken for a prolonged period at least 4-12 weeks to be of most benefit In disease like hepatitis you just use it by itself sometimes for months after this time you can consider adding Dandelion.

Used to increase milk production in mothers and for gallbladder problems.

Uses - Liver problems, gallbladder problems, hepatitis, to increase milk production.

Milk Thistle and Dandelion Together

Actions of Milk Thistle - Cholagogue, galactagogue, demulcent. Known as the liver regenerator.

Milk Thistle and dandelion together make a good and gentle liver cleanser, detoxifier and repairer. Use for liver or kidney damage, hepatitis (include Echinacea), jaundice, leptospirosis and parvo virus recovery. It may be helpful in chronic skin disorders, tumors and cancer. This is a major antioxidant. Pets that have been on a lot of veterinary drugs, heart worm prevention, vaccinations, de-worming drugs or chemotherapy need this healing from these herbs.

Motherwort

Actions - Sedative, emmenagogue, antispasmodic, cardiac tonic.

As its species name indicates, it has long been considered a nerve and heart remedy. It strengthens heart function, particularly where it is weak. Antispasmodic and sedative, the herb causes relaxation rather than drowsiness. Motherwort is considered a life giving plant, beneficial for all female disorders and a general heart tonic. Delayed or suppressed menses especially where anxiety or tension are involved, specific for over rapid heartbeat brought on by anxiety or tension, lowers high blood pressure and is used for the pains of birth and given for a few days after so as to prevent bleeding and infection.

Mullein

Actions - Expectorant, demulcent, mild diuretic, mild sedative, vulnerary.

The herb is famed for its powers in pulmonary ailments being much used in lung ailments of cattle, a bone flesh and cartilage builder, aids in healing respiratory ailments, asthma, bronchitis, sinus congestion, soothing to any inflammation and relieves pain, acts to relieve spasms and clears the lungs, tones mucous membranes of the respiratory system, inflammation of the trachea, painful coughs. The leaves of Mullein were traditionally fed to animals that cough especially horses.

Uses - Coughs, pneumonia, bronchitis, pleurisy, TB, asthma, diarrhea, internal bleeding of the lung and bowel.

Myrrh

Actions - Anti microbial, astringent, carminative, anti-catarrhal, expectorant, vulnerary, Antiseptic, antifungal, alterative.

Stimulates production of white blood cells and also has a good anti-microbial action so this is a good herb for immune boosting and fighting diseases.

Uses - Stomach viruses, coughs, asthma, infections of the mouth, mouth ulcers, gingivitis, sinusitis, laryngitis.

Externally - Healing and antiseptic to wounds and

abrasions.

Cautions - Use only in small amounts for short periods. Large amounts can speed heartbeat.

Nasturtium

Actions - Anti microbial, expectorant, anthelmintic.

The plant has a hot biting character especially in the seeds which were once used to make a popular pickle. Animals eat the whole plant greedily. The seeds of this plant are collected and used on poultry as a wormer. The seeds can be preserved in vinegar and used as a tonic and anti-worm remedy. A powerful anti-microbial especially when used locally on bacterial infections. Internally use for infections more so in the respiratory system such as bronchitis, flu and colds where it is used in breaking up congestion in the respiratory passages.

Uses - Bacterial infections, respiratory infections, as a tonic, poor sight, worms. Locally as a general antiseptic.

Neem

Actions - Anti-inflammatory, alterative, antibacterial, antiviral, antifungal, anthelmintic, bitter tonic, immune stimulant.

The name in Sanskrit means curer of all ailments and another name it is called is village pharmacy. Its antibacterial properties are good for Staph and Clostridia, Neem effectively kills lice and is good for topical applications to skin problems.

Uses - Ring worm, eczema , rash, arthritis and rheumatism and is used for malaria. Use as a wash for ticks, mites, scabies and fleas.

Cautions - Not for use for infants and the elderly and not for long term internal use.

Nettles

Actions - Astringent, diuretic, galactagogue, tonic, nutritive.

Nettle is perhaps best known as a highly nutritious feed herb/fodder for animals, and has been used through the ages for this purpose. It is considered a spring tonic and detoxifier for human and animal alike. One of the richest sources of chlorophyll in the vegetable kingdom, rich in iron, lime, sodium, Vit C, chlorine and contains much protein. Preventative against many ailments, increases milk yield, fattener for poultry. Good astringent for stopping bleeding anywhere but especially in the urinary tract. Good for eczema in the young especially in the nervous young. Good for pregnant and nursing mothers. The seeds can be used as a thyroid tonic.

Uses - Treatment of wasting diseases, poor appetite, lung disorders, blood impurities, worms, fever, cold, hay fever, allergies, eczema, diarrhea, hemorrhage.

Externally - Paralysis, rheumatism, arthritis, loss of muscular power.

Caution - Only buy the product prepared for herbal use.

Oats

Actions - Nerve tonic, anti-depressant, nutritive, demulcent, vulnerary.

Oats are a strength giving cereal low in starch high in mineral content especially potassium, phosphorus, magnesium and calcium and also the B vitamins. Is a nerve tonic and bone builder used for nervous debility, nervous exhaustion, general debility, skin conditions.

Uses - As a nutritive food, remedy and cure for rickets, important for strong teeth, hooves, horns, nails and hair.

Parsley

Actions - Diuretic, carminative, emmenagogue, expectorant.

Well-liked by sheep and goats, improves their milk yield and keeps them free from foot ills. It is a great enricher of the blood being very rich in iron and copper. Nutrient, digestive tract tonic, diuretic, high in potassium minerals and vitamins, bladder and kidney infections, incontinence, blood cleanser, immune builder, tonic for the blood vessels, aids in afterbirth pains, mainly used as a diuretic, carminative and emmenagogue. Is a good source of chlorophyll, parsley is useful for combating bad breath. Its diuretic properties are beneficial in: arthritic/rheumatic conditions associated with poor kidney function; urinary infections; kidney and bladder stones. Parsley also acts as a digestive tonic by easing spasms and minimizing flatulence.

Uses - Treatment of all disorders of the kidneys and bladder, gravel, stones, congestion, cystitis, jaundice, obesity, dropsy, worms, rheumatism, prostrate problems, sciatica, swellings of the joints, the root can be used for constipation and obstructions of the intestines.

Caution - Do not use in pregnancy.

Passion Flower Incarnata

Actions - Sedative, antispasmodic, anodyne, relaxant, epilepsy, shingles, asthma, hypotensive.

A good herb for insomnia and a very effective herb for nerve pains especially in conditions like shingles. This herbs focus is more on restlessness and irritability, hysteria and anxiety and is soothing to the mentally worried and overworked it acts on nervousness especially due to unrest, agitation, worry, exhaustion and cerebral excitement. Can be of benefit to horses that are generally nervous and apprehensive. Used in the treatment of convulsions, epilepsy, tremors, hypertension, nervous breakdowns, migraines and neuralgias.

Cautions - Large doses may cause nausea and vomiting. Do not use while pregnant.

Pau D'Arco

Actions - Alterative, anodyne, analgesic, antifungal,

antibacterial, anti-inflammatory, antioxidant, antiviral, diuretic, immune stimulant.

This herb comes from Brazil and is used by the Indians there. It possesses properties that are antibiotic, tumor inhibiting, virus killing, anti-fungal and anti-malarial. Builds up the immune system. It's anti-inflammatory action applies especially in the stomach and intestines as well as for conditions such as cystitis, inflammation of the cervix, arthritis and prostatitis, it is a good herb for fighting fungal infections while building up the immune system. This herb is used for lung, colon and prostrate cancer. It contains a chemical called lapachol that inhibits tumor cell growth by preventing them from metabolizing oxygen. Pau D'Arco also lowers blood sugar levels and acts as a mild laxative.

Pennyroyal

Actions - Carminative, diaphoretic, stimulant, emmenagogue, insecticide.

The forerunner of the cultivated mints, animals seek it for its tonic and stimulating properties, herdsmen use it after calving as a stimulant and restorative to the cow, abdominal colic due to wind, spasmodic pain, eases anxiety, its main use is as a emmenagogue to stimulate the menstrual process and strengthen uterine contractions. Helpful against nausea and nervous conditions.

Uses - Treatment of digestive ailments including failing appetite, sour stomach and internal gas, cough, pneumonia, fever, bronchitis and pleurisy, after birth exhaustion, female complaints.

Externally used as a insect repellant (oil) and a lotion for itching skin eg rashes, psoriasis etc.

Caution - Do not use in pregnancy or in large doses.

Peppermint

Actions - Carminative, diaphoretic, anti-spasmodic, anti-emetic, nervine, analgesic, anti-septic.

Best known for its ability to aid digestion and relieve gastrointestinal distress. Peppermint owes most of its medicinal value to menthol, which is cooling, anesthetic, antiseptic and soothing to the stomach. For horses, peppermint's aroma is useful for tempting fussy eaters and/or helping to mask the smell of less pleasant herbs in their feed. It eases flatulence/bloating, increases the flow of bile from the liver and relaxes both gastrointestinal spasms and tight skeletal muscles.

Uses- Nausea, heartburn, indigestion, colic, flatulence, dyspepsia, vomiting, fevers, migraine headaches and irritable bowel syndrome (IBS) and for travel sickness think of adding Ginger for this.

Caution - May reduce milk flow if breast feeding.

Plantain

Actions - Expectorant, demulcent, astringent, antibacterial, diuretic.

Goats and sheep enjoy its foliage and poultry seek out

the seeds. Plantain clears heat and removes excess fluid from the body while at the same time soothing inflammation and irritated tissues. The whole plant yields soothing mucilage similar to linseed, gentle expectorant while soothing sore and inflamed membranes, coughs, bronchitis etc. Its astringency aids in diarrhea and cystitis where there is bleeding. Is good for using in the treatment of stomach ulcers and has been used for blood poisoning. The plant is high in chlorophyll and good for use on wounds.

Uses - Treatment of dysentery, hemorrhages, internal obstructions and ulcers, fevers.

Externally - Wounds, sores, ulcers and all bites, eye disorders.

Poke Root - Phytolacca

Actions - Purgative, emetic, stimulant, anti-rheumatic and anti-catarrhal.

May be seen primarily as a remedy for use in infections of the upper respiratory tract removing catarrh and aiding in the cleansing of the lymphatic glands, it may be used for catarrh, tonsillitis, laryngitis and swollen glands. It will be found to be of value to problems elsewhere in the body involving the lymphatic system especially mastitis (Homoeopathic form works faster). Also used in long standing cases of rheumatism. Poke Root stimulates the immune system by increasing T cell activity. Care must be taken with this herb as in large doses it is a powerful emetic and purgative. Can be used as a lotion in mastitis. This herb in the past has been known as cancer root and has been used for breast cancer and tumors.

Uses - Mastitis and other lymphatic problems.

External Use - Breast cancer, tumors, mastitis, boils, fungal infections, shingles, psoriasis, scabies and eczema.

Cautions - This is a very strong herb so use it very carefully in small doses.

Raspberry

Actions - Astringent, tonic, refrigerant, parturient.

Raspberry leaf has been used for mares with oestrus problems and the attendant behavioral disturbances. For mares that have had or may have difficulty conceiving it can be given for a period prior to mating. Generally, raspberry leaf is used to tone the uterine muscles, encourage an easy labor, and hemorrhaging during and after birth

Highly tonic and cleansing improving the condition of the organism during pregnancy ensuring speedy and strong expulsion of the fetus at birth, use as a drench in retained afterbirth, acclaimed as a tonic for male animals and as a cure for sterility, becomes especially potent for female use when blended with feverfew - 3 parts to 1 part of feverfew. As a astringent it can be used in diarrhea and leucorrhoea, it is valuable in easing mouth problems such as mouth ulcers, bleeding gums and inflammations

Uses - Prevention and treatment of all female ailments, retained afterbirth, digestive ailments including diarrhea, treatment of mouth and throat ailments as a gargle.

Red Clover

Actions - Alterative, diuretic, expectorant, antispasmodic, nutritive.

The flowers are a powerful tonic and a cure for nervous twitches, wasting bodies and cough. The whole plant is sedative. Good for treating conditions like eczema and psoriasis and other chronic skin conditions. In the respiratory system we can use the actions of expectorant and antispasmodic to treat conditions such as bronchitis, whooping cough and maybe the eczema and asthma syndrome and as this herb seems to have a affinity for the throat we could use it for tonsillitis to. In the nervous system we can use the antispasmodic action to treat stress and nervousness along with hypertension. The alterative action of this herb helps to clean out the body and makes this herbs action on the skin very effective and it is probably this action that makes it useful in cancers especially breast and Ovary cancer. The herb has proved beneficial in cancers of the stomach and throat. This herb is in a lot of female formulas now because they extract the Isoflavones (Plant Hormones) from it and it is said to be very rich in these.

Uses - Tonic, treatment for general debility, weak nerves, throat ailments, cancers, tumors, detox, skin diseases and respiratory problems.

Rose Hips

Actions - Nutrient, mild laxative, mild diuretic, mild astringent.

The foliage is enjoyed by all animals. The flowers are tonic and astringent. The fruits are slightly aperient and rich in vitamin C. A good spring tonic and aid to general debility and exhaustion. Used to fight infection and curb stress. Rosehips are often fed to horses recuperating from injury as they help to restore the immune system and aid tissue repair and leaking capillaries with their bioflavonoids.

Rosemary

Actions - Carminative, aromatic, antispasmodic, anti-depressive, antiseptic, parasiticide.

It imparts a fine fragrance and tonic properties to the milk of goat and sheep which graze it eagerly. The powdered form is used on wounds as a antiseptic, nerve tonic, carminative, insecticide, acts as a circulatory and nerve stimulant, headache.

Uses - Treatment of all ailments of the heart, rheumatism, fits, epilepsy, paralysis, gastritis, diarrhea, dysentery.

Externally - Wounds, falling hair and nervous spasms.

Caution - Excessive large doses can poison and cause death.

Rue

Actions - Antispasmodic, emmenagogue, anti tussive, abortifacient.

The essential principal of the plant is Rutin which possesses most potent powers strengthening weakened blood vessels, toning the nerves and glands and imparting hardness to bones teeth and nails, highly antiseptic and is also a insecticide, it is also a old remedy for the prevention and cure of rabies. Regulates menses, used to bring on suppressed menses, the anti-spasmodic action is used to relax smooth muscles especially in the digestive system where it will ease gripping and bowel tension, spasmodic coughs, lowers elevated blood pressure.

Uses - Treatment of fevers, epilepsy, neuralgia, heart disease, ailments of the arteries and veins, worms, all skin parasites including scabies and ringworm,.

Caution - Avoid in pregnancy.

Reshi Mushroom

Actions - Immune stimulant, antibacterial, anti-tumor, adaptogen, rejuvenative, anti-inflammatory

As a immune stimulant it helps to activate the phagocytosis of macrophages and may increase interferon. Aids in the prevention of illness as well as in recovery. Helps normalize blood pressure reduces cholesterol and can inhibit histamine release. Inhibits the inflammation associated with allergies, bronchitis, conjunctivitis and rheumatism. Good for treating chronic hepatitis. Good for over overcoming fatigue, anxiety and stress while improving stamina at the same time.

Uses - Good as a all-round immune booster and restorative tonic. Works well with its fellow mushroom Shitake as they tend to complement each others actions and together they can be used to attack acute viral diseases. In chronic disease use 1/10 of the recommended dose.

Shitake Mushroom

Actions - Immune stimulant, antiviral, rejuvinative, aphrodisiac.

Animal studies have shown a antiviral and anti tumour activity as well as the stimulation of killer T cells. Shitake enhances the stem cells in the bone marrow to create more B and T cells. Lowers blood pressure by helping the body get rid of excessive salt and can be used in AIDs like diseases. Stimulates the production of interferon and provides significant protection against type A Viruses which causes epidemic influenza.

Uses - Good as a all-round immune booster and restorative tonic. Works well with its fellow mushroom Reshi as they tend to complement each others actions and together they can be used to attack acute viral diseases. In chronic disease use 1/10 of the recommended dose.

Sage

Actions - Carminative, antispasmodic, antiseptic, astringent.

Sage is well liked by animals and as with other aromatics makes the milk refreshing, tonic and increases the milk yield, it is a nervine, digestive and blood cleanser, a first rate remedy for all disorders of the throat, lungs and ears, inflamed and bleeding gums, inflamed tongue or general mouth inflammation, mouth ulcers, a good mouth wash.

Uses - Treatment of nerve debility, paralysis, all gastric ailments, constipation, obesity and female ailments, eczema, fevers, wound infections.

Dose - For horses infuse 1 teaspoon of powdered herb in 2 cups of water. Use in small doses. For sore mouths and throat ailments give mixed with honey.

Caution - Stimulates the muscles of the uterus so should be avoided during pregnancy.

Sarsaparilla

Actions - Alterative, diuretic, diaphoretic, anti-rheumatic, tonic.

Has a purifying effect on the genito urinary tract helping in the clearing of infections and the excretion of uric acid. Has chemicals and properties that aid in the production of testosterone, eliminates poisons and toxins from the blood and helps clean the system, useful in scaling skin conditions such as psoriasis, used in rheumatism and arthritis.

Uses - Rheumatism, arthritis, gout, skin eruptions, ringworm, internal inflammations, colds, catarrh.

Slippery Elm Bark Powder

Actions - Demulcent, emollient, nutrient, astringent. Slippery elm bark provides a nutritious gruel which also possesses remarkable medicinal properties acting as a poultice both internally and externally. A nutrient and food for very old or young or weak especially if mixed with honey, coats and heals all inflamed tissues internally and externally and is used for the stomach, intestines, ulcers, ulcerative colitis, enteritis, dysentery, constipation and internal bleeding of the digestive tract.

Uses - Treatment of all digestive complaints especially ulcers for which it is a specific, dysentery, all pectoral disorders including TB, lung and bronchial hemorrhage, wasting diseases, rickets, stunted growth. Calves with scour can be kept alive on this mixed with honey while the non treated can die.

Externally - A poultice for all skin ailments especially old ailments and hard swellings.

Shepherds Purse

Actions - Uterine stimulant, astringent, diuretic.
Possesses important astringent properties, all animals like this herb and poultry seek it eagerly.
A gentle diuretic, diarrhea, wounds, reduces

excessive menstruation.

Uses - Treatment of hemorrhages internal and external, profuse bleeding of deep wounds, kidney ailments, female problems.

Skullcap

Actions - Nervine tonic, sedative, antispasmodic.
Supreme nerve herb and has restored many cases of nervous disorders, nervous tension, seizures, epilepsy, PMS, carminative nervine and nervous system repairer, pain reliever, spinal problems, twitching muscles, rheumatism, high blood pressure, restlessness, nervous heart conditions.

Uses - Treatment of all nervous complaints especially hysteria, fits, meningitis, nervous spasms, gastroenteritis, an old cure for rabies.

St Johns Wort see Hypericum

Sweet Violets

Actions - Alterative, expectorant, anti-inflammatory, anti-cancer, diuretic, antifungal, antiseptic.
Is used with Red Clover as a detoxifier and a blood cleanser. Especially useful to animals that have had a toxic reaction to Vaccination. Good for coughs and bronchitis. Can be used as a poultice on cancer tumors.

Uses - Skin problems, tumors, warts, behavior reactions or other aggravations from vaccination, digestive disorders, seizures, cancer, cysts, boils, abscesses, chronic skin diseases.

Senna Pods

Actions - Cathartic

One of the most important laxatives because it is also a cleanser and restorative of the entire digestive system. The griping tendency is diminished by the addition of powdered ginger. As heat destroy the properties of this herb it should be prepared as a cold water infusion steeping the pods or leaves for a minimum of 4 hours.

Uses - Treatment of constipation.

Dose - 24 large senna pods for cows. Soak in cold water for a minimum of 4 hours but preferably 7 hours. Add half a teaspoon of ginger to 20 to 24. Give the dose last thing at night at least 2 hours after food has been taken.

Tansy

Actions - Digestive bitter, carminative, emmenagogue, vermifuge, anthelmintic.

Cows and sheep eat the herb, powerful worm expellant, effective against round worm and thread worm and may be used in children as a enema, as a bitter it will stimulate the digestive process, eases dyspepsia, stimulate menses.

Uses - Treatment of all types of worms, debility, causes abortion.

Caution - Avoid during Pregnancy.

Tea Tree Oil

Australian Tea Tree Oil is one of the world's best antiseptics and is also anti-bacterial, anti-fungal and anti-viral which means you can use it with good results on virtually any wound on the skin.
Use for external applications.

Thyme

Actions - Carminative, antimicrobial, antispasmodic, expectorant, astringent, anthelmintic.
Eaten by sheep and goats and is a milk tonic for them, the whole herb is tonic and antiseptic, A favorite Bee herb and should be planted by all apiaries, can be used for digestive or respiratory infections, use as a gargle for laryngitis or tonsillitis, eases sore throats and coughs, bronchitis, whooping cough, asthma, diarrhea and dyspepsia and sluggish digestion,
Uses - Treatment of all digestive complaints including colic, inflammation of the liver, rickets, all pectoral ailments, hysteria, nervousness, sciatica, retention of afterbirth, inflamed or diseased uterus, metritis, worms including hook worm.

Valerian

Actions - Sedative, antispasmodic, hypnotic, hypotensive, carminative.
A powerful nervine and sedative stronger than other

herbal sedatives, pain reliever, reduces anxiety, hysteria, soothes the nervous system, reduces high blood pressure, slows and strengthens the heart and calms palpitations, useful for muscle spasms, arthritic pain, spinal injuries, aids indigestion and gas, insomnia, cramps, colic, can help with migraines. Valerian root is one of the most widely used herbal nervines for calming horses as it can relieve anxiety and excitability without reducing the horse's mental faculties or their physical ability to perform.

Uses - Treatment of epilepsy, hysteria, acute constipation, worms, malaria, pain and for sensitive nervous animals.

Externally - The oil is used as a rub for paralyzed limbs, cramps, swollen arteries and veins.

Caution - Do not mix with drug tranquillizers.

Vervain

Actions - Nerve tonic, hepatic, sedative, antispasmodic, diaphoretic.

A favorite of Hippocrates, valuable in every type of fever use in the early stages, nervous disorders, eye problems, plague remedy of ancient times, strengthens the nervous system while relaxing any tension or stress, depression especially if it comes on after a illness, seizures, hysteria, inflammation of the gallbladder, jaundice, use as a mouth wash in gum disease.

Uses - Treatments of all fevers , fits, convulsions,

hysteria, liver complaints, gallstones.

Externally - Weak and inflamed eyes, inflamed throats, sore and ulcerated mouths.

Wild Yam

Actions - Antispasmodic, anti-inflammatory, anti-rheumatic,

The first birth control pills were once based on this remedy. Used for severe digestive pain in conditions such as colic, dysmenorrhea, and ovarian and uterine pains. Also used in the treatment of rheumatoid arthritis especially when there is painful inflammation. Muscle cramps and spasms, nerve pains and threatened miscarriage.

Dose - For horses 1 tablespoon of powder twice daily.

Willow Bark (White Willow)

Actions - Febrifuge ,bitter tonic, astringent, antiseptic, analgesic, anti-inflammatory, anti-rheumatic.

Willow Bark can be thought of as caveman's Aspirin as it was developed from this. Cattle and horses eat the young shoots and foliage. It is a refrigerant herb valuable in fevers and pain relief but can take a while to get into the system so think of looking for results especially in pain in about a days time.

Uses - Treatment of all fevers, debility, enteritis, colic, pleurisy, rheumatism, sciatica and urinary

infections as the excretion of salicylic acid in urine soothes a inflamed tract.
Externally - Rickets and cramp.

Witch Hazel

Actions - Astringent one of the most widely used ones. Antiseptic.

As with all astringents this herb may be used wherever there is bleeding both externally and internally, commonly used for piles, bruises and inflamed swellings, varicose veins, diarrhea.

Uses - Internally to heal ulcerated and burnt tissues in cases of poisoning, stomach and intestinal ulcers, Externally - wounds, sores, bruises, ulcers, inflammation of the organs of reproduction, torn udders resulting in milk leakage, inflamed udders and glands, sore eyes and inflamed ears.

Withania (Ashwagandha)

Actions - Adaptogen, analgesic, anti-tumor, hormone regulator, pregnancy tonic, rejuvinative.

This herb is a pregnancy tonic for both the foetus and a weak mother, relieves pain by lowering serotonin levels which contribute to the sensitivity of pain receptors in the body. Good for debility, nervous exhaustion especially due to stress and chronic diseases especially those marked by inflammation. Retards various aspects of the aging process and increases stamina and also sexual desire.

Wood Betony

Actions - Alterative, analgesic, antispasmodic, astringent, Bitter tonic, sedative, circulatory stimulant, diuretic.

Juliette de Bairacli Levy says the whole plant possesses a pungent and peculiar aroma especially when trampled on. This would show the plant to have a high oil content. Was once used as a smoke and snuff to treat headaches. Wood Betony is used for severe pains in the face and head consider it for horses with severe sinus or those who always toss there head.

Uses - Treatment of debility, gastritis, diarrhea, acidity, glandular deficiency, arthritis, rheumatism, exhaustion, sciatica, hypertension, kidney dysfunction.

Externally - arthritis, rheumatism, sciatica, rickets, tumors, swellings, boils, abscesses, corns, warts and blisters, gingivitis, as a poultice to draw out splinters and boils.

Wormwood

Actions - Bitter tonic, carminative, anthelmintic, anti-inflammatory.

The foliage is eaten by horses, cows and sheep. Its chief merits are worm expellant (round worm and pinworm) and tonic. A important herb for female ailments, protects against contagious diseases and plagues, insecticide, hair tonic, as a bitter it stimulates the digestive process, fevers, infections.

Uses - Treatment of all worms, failing appetite, gastritis, gastric ulcers,, acidity, enteritis, constipation, jaundice, TB, tumor, pneumonia, pleurisy, all female ailments and bladder problems.

Externally - Prevention of falling hair, insecticide especially lice, sores, mange, inflammation of the ear, conjunctivitis.

Yarrow

Actions - Diaphoretic, astringent, diuretic, antiseptic, hypotensive.

It is a famed wound herb for staunching excess bleeding and derives it name from the Greek Warrior Achilles who healed his wounds and those of his soldiers with yarrow blossoms.

The herb is one of the best diaphoretics known to herbalists opening the skin pores and inducing lavish perspiration, sheep seek out the herb on dry ground as a food tonic, fevers, as a urinary antiseptic it can be used for cystitis, specific in thrombotic conditions associated with high blood pressure.

Uses - Treatment of all fevers, pneumonia, pleurisy, inflamed throat, hemorrhages, uterine hemorrhages, dysentery, hysteria, epilepsy, rheumatism, colic.

Externally - Wounds, skin eruptions, abscess, earache.

Yellow Dock

Actions - Alterative, Cholagogue, purgative, mild astringent.

A powerful blood purifier and astringent. It is used in treating all diseases of the blood and skin. Very high in iron, making it useful for treating anemia. It nourishes and detoxifies the liver and cleanses and enriches the blood.

Used extensively for skin complaints such as psoriasis, a mild acting remedy for the relief of constipation, has a action on the gallbladder.

Uses - Constipation, skin problems, gallbladder problems, jaundice.

Dose - For horses 1 tablespoon of powder twice daily, less if purgative action is to much.

Yucca

Actions - Alterative, anti-inflammatory, anti-rheumatic, laxative.

This herb is gaining attention for its treatment in dogs for arthritis, hip displasia and other degenerative hip and bone diseases. It seems to have a natural anti-inflammatory effect on the body. The saponins in Yucca mimic the structure and effects of cortisone.

Also aids in digestion and is a blood cleanser. Is now being used for gout.

Cautions - Use only the dried root. Long time use may impair the assimilation of the fat soluble vitamins.

Homeopathic Supplement

Homeopathy has been around now for hundreds of years and unlike most other forms of medicine its rules have not changed and will not for they are based on a essential truth. The main rule is Like cures Like or if we break down the word Homeopathy homo means the same and pathy means disease. As Homoeopathy is a very hard science to learn and as it kind of sits or balances on the border of hard science and metaphysics I will not try to explain to you what it is here as it would probably take a whole book to do this but I will say this, in the UK and a lot of countries in Europe it is on and paid for by the National Health System and anything that can get a politician to open their purse must work.

It is said that Homeopathy sits on a three legged stool. What this means is that if a remedy has at least three symptoms in the same strength as the symptoms you are trying to match then that remedy is a potential cure for your condition or if not cure it will offer the condition relief. The more symptoms you can match to the remedy the better the remedy will work for the rule is likes cure likes not vaguely similar cures. Listed below are some common Homoeopathic Remedies and some of the symptoms they cover. The idea is to find one remedy that covers most of your symptoms. To make the remedies as closer a match as we can we ask lots of questions like the ones below and after we gather all the answers we have what is called a good Symptom Picture which we then try to match as accurately as we can to a Remedy. Most Homeopathic Materia Medicas are set out to answer the questions listed below with the mind symptoms being the most important. Questions on time, position and temperature are good for making a choice between to very close remedies. The best Materia Medica for the lay person is Boerickes and you should be able to view this on a few Homeopathic websites.

Symptom Guide Questions

1. Was there a sudden onset of the condition, at what time?
2. What time of the day does the patient feel either better or worse.
3. What is the effect of motion? jarring? walking? running?
4. What is the effect of drinking fluids? warm and or cold drinks?
5. Is the patient thirsty or not at all? sips or gulps?
6. Is the onset from exertion? overeating? weather changes? emotions?
7. Mental emotional state of patient?
8. Better warm room? warm air?
9. Better cool room? cool open air?
10 Are the respirations upper chest movements or in the abdomen?
11 Respirations - dry or wet?
12 Expectoration - watery or stringy mucous, easy or difficult.

13   Is there coughing

14   Position - better or worse from sitting? standing? lying? lying on which side?

15   Along with the condition is there fever? gas? belching? wind?

Modality - The questions above are covering what the Homoeopaths call modalities which basically mean are covering a condition that makes the patient better or worse. I will list the main Modalities below. The Modalities help us to distinguish which remedy is right for the case especially when we have a group that look as though they may all work which is what I am giving you und the disease heading. Using modalities forces you to think what really is going on, is this the nature of the beast or the nature of the disease.

Time - Better or Worse morning, night, weekly, monthly, seasonally etc.

Motion - Better or Worse first movement, rest, exertion, walking, stretching, rising up etc

Temperature - Better or Worse heat, cold, cold air blowing, sudden change etc.

Body Activity - Better or Worse eating, drinking, urinating, defecating, sleep, coughing etc

Weather - - Better or Worse, damp, sunny, foggy, storms, sudden changes etc.

Senses - Better or Worse - touch, pressure, noise, light, odors etc.

Position - Better or Worse lying, standing, sitting,

stretched out, doubled up, right side etc.

Mind - Excitement, anger, fear, stress, better busy, nervous all the time etc.

Now read through all the remedies in the Marteria Medica (Homoeopathic Remedy Reference) and you will notice that most of them have Mind or mental symptoms kind of describing the personalities or moods a good example is Nux Vomica, I think we all know a nasty type of individual that this remedy would be suited to and meaning as though the individual is suited to this remedy then the remedy would have a curative action on them but don't expect it to change the nature of the beast. One of the main rules of Homeopathy is the closer the match of the remedy the higher the Potency you use but if you are not used to Homoeopathy just use the 30C potency and remember what I said about the 3 legged stool. Potency is a measure of strength and depth of action.

Remember as mentioned before Homoeopathy sits on a three legged stool. What this means is that if a remedy has at least three symptoms in the same strength as your symptoms then that remedy is a potential cure.

Note - The best prescribing guide for the layman is **Boerickes Materia Medica With Repertory.**

Another good guide is **The Complete Book Of Homeopathy by Dr Michael Weiner.**

I always buy my books on Homeopathy from India as they are quarter the price and there is always a wide selection. Put B. Jain Publishers into the google search engine go to their web site and check out these books and I am sure you will be pleased with what you find.

Disease Nosodes

Nosodes are remedies made from disease material mainly from the tissues, discharges, exudates, excretions, suppurations or secretions of a infected being. Simply stated a Nosode is a homeopathic remedy prepared from a pathological specimen. Rabies Nosode, for example starts with the saliva of a rabid dog and is then potentized.

Nosodes have many uses and are widely used in homeopathic practice to help limit cases of infectious diseases and to help during the recovery phase of a disease especially the ones that linger and drag on. There are Nosodes for most infectious diseases of animals and humans the use of Nosodes in this way is referred to as isopathy rather than Homoeopathy. They are often used in farm situations, to limit the spread and the effects of infectious diseases. This has especially been used as a vital component of mastitis control on many farms, both organic and conventional. One documented event about Nosodes dates back to Napoleon marching his Legions through Europe and spreading Typhoid in their wake, the towns that had the best cure rates were the ones where the local Homoeopaths used a Nosode of the disease.

Nosodes can be used in the prevention of infectious

diseases in the manner of vaccination but they work by a completely different mechanism then from the raising of antibodies that vaccines work by. As yet it is not actually known how they work but they have survived hundreds of years ridicule by producing results and will carry on doing so.

The best known study into Nosodes was done by Dr. Christopher Day of England involving 'kennel cough' in a boarding kennel. At the time he was called in, there were 40 dogs in the kennel with 35 that had kennel cough. About half had been vaccinated for this malady. He gave a Nosode to all the animals that were there and all the dogs that came in through the rest of the summer, which was another 214 dogs. He successfully reduced the incidence of kennel cough from over 90% to less than 2%.

Nosodes used for the prevention of diseases are usually given in the 30C potency. A good dosing regime is one dose given night and morning for 3 days followed by one per month for the next 6 months. This generally provides a good level of protection after the first week. A good example of how this can be used is a puppy given the Nosode of Parvovirus at 3 to 4 weeks of age instead of having to wait for 9 weeks for the vaccination, this way the puppy is protected before given the vaccination.

Nosodes can have homeopathic therapeutic properties in their own right. Such Nosodes are found in the Homoeopathic Materia Medica and have undergone a proper 'proving'. Examples are Bacillinum, Carcinosinum, Medorrhinum, Psorinum,

Tuberculinum.

Dose - Dr. Surjit S. Makker recommends 20ml of remedy mixed with 8 liters of water for 100 birds. This medicated water should be shaken well and put in drinkers accordingly. For individual birds give them 2-3 pellets by mouth and keep them calm.

Notes

Materia Medica

Note - All Homeopathic Remedies are given in Potency and not in material Form.

Aconite

Characteristics - Aconite is best used in the first stages of a illness, especially when fear and anxiety are present. Symptoms appear suddenly, without warning and they may be caused by exposure to cold winds or draughts or by a severe fright. Symptoms are a marked restlessness, animal displays extreme anxiety or fear, high fever with a burning skin, extreme sweating and a burning thirst, a hoarse dry painful cough, bright light noises stress and cold worsen the symptoms, rest and quiet relieves the symptoms. The pains of Aconite are unbearable, sharp, shooting, burning pains, tingling and numbness. A remedy for fevers and inflammatory states, use at the first sign of all fevers, shivering with cold sweats, difficult breathing, animal shows desire for large quantities of water, symptoms worse at midnight, symptoms improve in the open air.

Mind - Great fear, anxiety, restlessness, extreme sensitivity to pain, worry, foreboding.

Better - In open air, warmth, rest.

Worse - In the evening and night, particularly before midnight, lying on affected side.

Allium Cepa

Characteristics - Increased secretions from the eyes and nose, like those of the common cold. Frequent sneezing with watery discharge which burns the nose and upper lip, but the eye discharge is bland and doesn't burn (the opposite of Euphrasia). Tickling in the throat with incessant cough (feels as if larynx is split) holds throat when coughing. Being in cool open air relieves the symptoms, eyelids are swollen and red, abdominal tympany with wind, this remedy is indicated in the early stages of most catarrhal conditions, mild forms of cat flu can be cut short if given early.

Better - Cold room (except cough), open air.

Worse - Evening, warm room, odors.

Antimonium Tartaricum - Ant Tart

Characteristics - Is characterized by a loose rattling unproductive cough such as is often herd in cats. Respiration can be very difficult with much gasping. There is usually thirst for little and often. Symptoms are worse in the evening, lying down and in cold damp weather or a warm room. Confined largely to respiratory diseases, abundant bronchial secretions, great rattling of mucous with little expectoration, drowsiness, debility and sweat.

Mind - Drowsy and despondent, fear of being alone, child will not be touched without whining.

Better - Sitting erect, from burping and expectoration.

Worse - Evenings, lying down, damp cold weather.

Apis

Characteristics - Apis is used for various types of swelling and inflammation such as that from animal bites and bites and stings from insects, it is also used for measles, mumps, sore throats, sore red eyes and fever. Apis is a quick acting remedy for inflammations especially those ones with edema and lots of swelling which is its main use. Acute nephritis with scanty and burning urine there may be some blood in the urine. . Symptoms are swelling with edema which makes the effected parts look shiny, red and puffy, the swollen parts feel soggy and waterlogged, a fever that develops rapidly but without thirst, extreme restlessness and fidgeting, an irritable nature and perhaps jealous, cool air and cold compresses relieve the symptoms. Pains are burning and stinging, arthritis with swelling, animals seek cold surface to lie on, swollen eyelids, may be swollen ears, may be blood in the urine, in the horse and cow there may be edema in the lower limbs while in dogs abdominal dropsy is seen. Symptoms get worse from heat and improve in the open air and from cold bathing.

Mind - Apathy, indifference, awkward.

Better - By cold, (room, air or application)

Worse - From warmth, pressure, late in the afternoon, from sleeping.

Arnica

Characteristics - Bruises and similar injuries where the skin is unbroken and there is mental or emotional shock. Symptoms are any type of bruising or similar injury caused by crushing, squeezing or wrenching, muscles strains which feel sore and bruised, shock after accidents, there is a fear of being touched because of the pain, good for the soreness after birth and medical operations.

Arnica can be used in potency and also as a cream. The cream must not be used on broken skin or wounds. Animal shrinks away when you try to touch it, symptoms improve when lying down.

Mind - Fears touch or approach, whole body oversensitive.

Better - Lying down or with head low.

Worse - Least touch, motion, damp and cold.

Arsenic Album

Characteristics - Burning pains relieved by heat, anxious, restless, weak and chilly with an air of fear and hopelessness. Anxiety or restlessness are often present where this remedy is indicated. Discharge from eyes and nose are watery and acrid causing ulceration in those regions. The mouth is usually dry and the patient is usually thirsty. Dramatic vomiting and diarrhea often simultaneously indicate its use if the modalities agree. The patient may have wheezing respiration and allergic asthmatic conditions can respond well. The skin can be dry, scaly and scruffy. Symptoms are worse for cold and wet better for warmth. Tries to find relief in motion but immediately feels weak with movement. Restless, feels cold, complains of general weakness, discharges burn the skin.

Mind - Fear with despair and restlessness.

Better - Warmth, open air, relieved by sweat, hot drinks, lying down (but restless).

Worse - Cold air, after midnight eg 1 to 3am. Wet damp weather and near sea shore.

Belladonna

Characteristics - This is one of the great fever remedies, conditions requiring its use usually being of violent and sudden onset. Heat, redness, pain and swelling characterize its symptoms. It is one of the main remedies used in convulsions. Pupils are usually dilated which is a keynote for this remedy. Acute ear inflammation where there is heat, pain and swelling respond well. The mouth is usually dry and there is great thirst. With Belladonna always think BIRDS. B for burning, I for irritability, R for redness, D for delirium and S for spasms.

Mind - Hallucinations, delirium, rages, bites, strikes, desire to escape.

Better - For quiet, dark, rest with slight warmth.

Worse - For noise, touch or jarring motion.

Bellis Perennis

Characteristics - Trauma to abdomen and pelvic organs especially after surgery and child birth if arnica does not give relief. Injuries to the nerves with intense soreness, back ache from hard physical work such as gardening, pain is bruised sore and aching, better cold presses, worse touch, after getting wet.

The animal is unwilling to move and when made to do so evinces pain, muscular stiffness is prominent.

Worse - Left side and cold wind.

Bryonia

Characteristics - This remedy shows both diarrhea and constipation symptoms, the latter usually in chronic conditions. The mouth is often dry and there is great thirst. The tongue is often coated yellow. It is of great help in many cases of rheumatism or arthritis where the symptoms agree. There is often respiratory signs with a hoarse hacking cough. All symptoms are worse for movement and better for rest.

Mind - Irritable, delirium.

Better - Lying on the painful side, pressure, rest and cold things.

Worse - Warmth, motion, morning, eating and touch.

Calendula

Characteristics - The part used is the Flowers and it is used for wounds and skin irritations, it is healing, soothing, anti-inflammatory, astringent, anti-fungal and anti-microbial.

Use as a lotion for cuts, grazes, infected sores, fungal infections, any skin inflammations, regulates the oil production of the skin so is good for acne, to stop bleeding, for bruises and sprains, skin ulcers and minor burns and scolds.

Note - The tincture of this is used as a lotion diluted at 1 to 10.

Cantharis

Characteristics - Important first aid remedy for minor burns and for other pains that feel burning and fiery, also has a healing effect on the bladder, urethra and other parts of the urinary tract where burning pain is the key symptom, burns and scalds especially where blistering and inflammation occur, sunburn, insect bites that feel hot and burn, cystitis. Pains are violent burning, cutting, stabbing or smarting, rawness, use when the animal appears distressed when passing urine, or tries to pass and cannot. Better from warmth rest and rubbing.

Mind - Furious delirium, acute mania generally of a sexual type, crying, barking.

Better - From rubbing

Worse - From touch or approach, from urinating,

from drinking cold water.

Carbo Vegetabilis

Characteristics - Patient exhibits mental and physical sluggishness and symptoms come on slowly, generalized weakness of all functions especially digestion, overweight, torpid, lazy, complaints of coldness, pains usually described as burning, pressing pains, wishes to be fanned, digestive problems such as belching often accompany any illness.

Mind - Aversion to darkness, sudden loss of memory.

Better - Being fanned, passing gas, rest.

Worse - Morning and evening, exertion, cold, tight clothes at abdomen.

Causticum

Characteristics - Burns and burning pains such as cystitis also used for dry coughs, burns to the skin especially with marked inflammation and blistering, coughs, laryngitis and hoarseness from straining and over using voice, cystitis especially with involuntary passing of urine when coughing, chronic cystitis, exposure to cold dry air may make symptoms worse.

Mind - Least thing makes it cry, sad, hopeless. Ailments from long lasting grief.

Better - In damp wet weather, warmth.

Worse - Cold winds.

Euphrasia

Characteristics - Affects the mucous membranes of the eyes, nose and chest producing copious watery secretions,eye secretions cause smarting of the skin while the nose discharge is bland. Used for conjunctivitis, eye strain generally but especially from computers, eyes that feel sore and inflamed and look red, hay fever symptoms including a tickly throat, sneezing, a runny nose, and itchy red watering eyes. Sunlight wind and warmth worsen the symptoms. Use for Dogs who have had their head out of the window for too long, symptoms better in dim light or darkness, in all species a tendency to diarrhea occurs.

Better - In the dark

Worse - From light, indoors, in the evening.

Hypericum

Characteristics - Used for bruises and other injuries especially to nerve rich areas like the fingers, lips, ears, eyes ,tail bone, good for the pain of puncture wounds of any cause eg animal or insect. Helps with the pains after operations especially amputations. Pains are violent shooting pains along a nerve path, burning, tingling and numbness. Worse from shock and touch and better from rubbing, horse fly bites, symptoms worse cold better warmth.

Mind - Anxiety, melancholy, effects of shock.

Better - Bending head backward.

Worse - Cold, dampness and touch.

Ipecac

Characteristics - Indicated for complaints of persistent nausea not relieved by vomiting, ailments caused by eating rich or indigestible type of foods such as ice-cream, sweets etc., useful to stop bleeding if blood is bright red.

Mind - Easily irritated, child cries or screams continuously, wanting something but not sure what they desire, holds everything in contempt.

Worse - Warm, moist weather, lying down.

Kali Bichromicum

Characteristics - Has a affinity for the mucous membranes of the body, tough stringy viscid secretions sometimes forming thick yellow green mucous, sinus infections, suited for fleshy fat light complexioned people, general weakness.

Better - Heat

Worse - Cold, beer, morning, undressing.

Kali Carbonicum

Characteristics - Has a affinity for the mucous membranes digestive and respiratory, very tired, anemic, flabby tissues which may be swollen, sweat, backache, weakness, many conditions have a aggravation at 2am to 4am, often stays immobile when ill.

Mind - Very irritable, hypersensitive to pain, despondent.

Better - During the day, sitting down, bending forward, warmth.

Worse - Cold weather, between 2am and 4am.

Lachesis

Characteristics - Many symptoms tend to be left sided, cannot bear tight clothing, symptoms worse on awakening, symptoms relieved with onset of the menstrual flow. Short dry cough, feels relief after coughing up watery phlegm, feeling of constriction in throat and chest, better bending forward.

Mind - Overly talkative, impatient, sad, jealous, no desire to mix with world.

Better - Release of pressure, eating fruit, cold, discharges.

Worse - Pressure, touch, after sleep, heat, hot weather.

Ledum

Characteristics - Has a action on the capillaries and is useful for cleaning up bruises especially around the eyes, mainly used for puncture wounds made by sharp points such as nails and wood splinters and insect bites and stings especially ones that don't heal properly and look blue and puffy. Wounds that feel cold to the touch, septic conditions, sprains, pains are throbbing, tearing ,prickling, they shoot upwards, stiff and sore. Better cold, cold bathing. This remedy was used in the past along with hypericum to ward off tetanus especially in deep wounds

Better - From cold.

Worse - At night and from heat.

Lycopodium

Characteristics - Exerts most of its effects on the digestive organs, liver, kidneys and respiratory systems. The patient dislikes being left alone and appears apprehensive. The nose is often blocked and there may be blisters on the tongue. Eating a little food always satisfies the appetite but appetite is very marked. The belly is usually bloated. The stool appears hard and small and is expelled only with difficulty accompanied by ineffectual straining. Urination is also a slow process and the urine has a red sediment. Symptoms are worse for heat generally and better for cold.

Mind - Melancholy, afraid to be alone, apprehensive.

Better - By motion, on getting cold.

Worse - From heat.

Natrum Sulphuricum

Characteristics - A good liver remedy, emotional and mental difficulties arising after head injury, useful in problems associated with rainy weather and dampness, patient feels every change from dry to wet weather, may remove excess water and fluid retention from the body.

Mind - Lively music saddens, melancholy, inability to think, dislikes to speak or be spoken to.

Better - Dry weather and environments, pressure, change of position.

Worse - Damp weather, damp basements, lying on left side.

Nux Vom

Characteristics - The remedy for overindulgence, adapted especially to thin irritable energetic people who attend with great detail to tasks, quarrelsome, nervous, intelligent, hypochondriacal, oversensitive to noise music and light, craves stimulants.

Primarily used in the digestive sphere, its greatest reputation is in helping disturbances following overeating of unsuitable foods. Feces is usually hard but diarrhea can follow overeating. There is abdominal discomfort, flatulence, irritability and sensitivity to noise. Symptoms are generally worse for noise and better after rest or for damp weather.

Mind - Very irritable, sensitive to all impressions, malicious, disposed to reproach others.

Better - Wet weather, lying down, uninterrupted nap.

Worse - Overeating, mental over exertion, sensory stimulation ie sound, sight, touch etc.

Phosphorus

Characteristics - Irritated and inflamed mucous and serous membranes are the key feature of this remedy. Is a very sudden remedy with suddenness of symptoms. The patient is sensitive to loud and sudden noises (eg thunder fireworks etc). Degenerative processes and bone destruction respond well to Phosphorus. Food is suddenly vomited back up when it has been warmed in the stomach, gums can be ulcerated and bloody. Hepatitis, jaundice, pancreatic disease and nephritis come into its sphere. Urine may be bloody. A very painful cough is also a symptom. Wounds that perpetually bleed may also be helped. The patient is usually in poor body condition. Symptoms are worse for touch, exertion, in the evening and during thunder storm. Better for cold and sleep.

Mind - Low spirits, restless, fidgety.

Better - In the dark, lying on the right side, from the cold, sleep.

Worse - Touch, from exertion and in the evening.

Pulsatilla

Characteristics - Often indicated for those with mild, gentle, timid yielding dispositions who are easily moved to laughter and tears, The Pulsatilla person wants to be held and loved, moods changeable and fickle, the patient is chilly but desires strolling in cold air, symptoms are erratic and change frequently, pains are wandering, pains that grow gradually in intensity, fever without thirst despite dry mouth, bland yellow discharges.

Mind - Weeps easily, timid, fears to be alone - dark - ghosts, likes sympathy and fuss, highly emotional, easily discouraged, sensitive.

Better - Open air, cold applications, consolation relieves symptoms.

Worse - Evening before midnight, warmth, after eating fat rich food.

Rhus Tox

Characteristics - Is the most famous of the rheumatic remedies. The skin and muscular skeletal system are its main spheres. Small red papules in the skin and sometimes vesicles are typical lesions with much scratching. In all cases of damage to muscles think of Rhus and the symptoms of arthritis which are worse after rest particularly if this follows strenuous exertion. The symptoms improve with limbering up , The worst pains are seen as the animal arises from its bed.

Mind - Listless, sad, extreme restlessness, great apprehension at night.

Better - Warmth, walking, from stretching out limbs.

Worse - During sleep, cold wet rainy weather and at night.

Ruta

Characteristics - Has effects on the joints, tendons, cartilages, and the periosteum which is a fine membrane that covers bones and gives it that shiny look, it is also used for eye strain where the vision goes dim.

Used for painful bruises affecting the bones, dislocations, strains to the tendons or joints, aching with restlessness, pains are gnawing, digging, burning, bruised, sore as if beaten, bones as if broken, pain deep in the bones, rheumatism.

Better - From lying and warmth.

Worse - From over exertion, touch, cold wet weather.

Silica

Characteristics - Fits the shy chilly patient who is reluctant to enter the room, chronic inflammatory conditions such as sinus, helps in the removal of foreign bodies such as splinters and seeds, ripens abscesses, ailments attended with pus formation. Use silica and be prepared to use it for a while sometimes up to 3 weeks.

Mind - Faint hearted, anxious, yielding.

Better - Warmth, wet or humid weather.

Worse - Morning, from lying down, cold.

Staphysagria

Characteristics - Suits sensitive people who suppress their feelings and suffer in silence or who boil over with indignation, remedy for cuts and wounds especially those that are from medical procedures and have the mentioned feelings. Nervous states of animals. The pains are stinging, stitching, smarting, squeezing, as if stabbed by a knife. Worse from touch, emotions and suppressed anger.

Better - Warmth, rest at night.

Worse - Touch on affected parts, loss of fluids.

Symphytum

Characteristics - Causes bone to grow and promotes fast healing should be given for all fractures. Used for injuries to the hard parts of the body while arnica is for the soft parts. Also used for eye injuries caused from blows.

Caution - do not use if a pin has been placed in the bone as the pin has to be removed latter.

Tarentula Cubensis

Characteristics - For abscesses, boils, carbuncles, swellings of any kind but especially on the back of the neck where the skin turns black, red/blue or purple with great pain. Deep septic conditions with hardening of the effected part, condition comes on fast, pains are burning, stinging, throbbing, pricking like a needle.

Worse - Night.

Urtica Urens

Characteristics - Can be used for burns and also for cystitis where the urine burns the skin and there is dificulty passing urine. Symptoms are stinging pains, swellings particularly blistery swellings, itching.

Worse - Cool moist air, touch.

Vitamin C

Vitamin C is the primary antioxidant in the lungs and a powerful antihistamine without side effects. Low vitamin C dramatically increases histamine levels which put you at greater risks for inflammation responses in the body. Always give a high dose of Vitamin C to animals before any operation where they require a anesthetic for the reasons mentioned above as they will recover faster and better from the anesthetic and maybe the inflammation from the surgical incisions will be toned down a bit.

Vitamin C is needed by the immune system and is necessary for healing and the prevention of infections along with being a potent antioxidant with anti-bacterial and antiviral actions. It is also essential for the utilization of the essential amino acids lysine (anti-viral) and proline. Another point to consider is that stress depletes the body's supply of Vitamin C so this may be another factor in the cause of many diseases. Vit C is essential for the formation of collagen tissue which is vital in tendons and cartilage so always consider this in muscle and back injuries and especially trauma injuries.

Sodium Ascorbate is good for use on animals as it is virtually tasteless when added to the animal's food and does not curdle milk. This can be used in high doses when needed for example dose till the bowels become loose then back the dose off. For severe situations you can use a injectable Vitamin C, in Australia we use Troys Injectable Vit C which we get from the Agricultural Stock Feed Shops or Co Ops. Use a large gauge needle with this as some animals have rather thick hides and the liquid solution is also fairly thick.

Think of using Vitamin C in all operations and all acute diseases. It is a good last resort to think of before the rifle especially in the deadly acute diseases where as a last resort you would use the injectable form in a intramuscular injection, this can also be a good gauge as to what may happen as these injections hurt like hell so if the animal turns around and gives you a filthy look then there is a good chance that they may live and if they do not seem to notice the injection well the chances don't look too good. So remember always keep a bottle of Injectable C in the fridge for emergencies.

Good Herb Sources Of Vitamin C

Alfalfa, Burdock, Catnip, Cayenne, Chickweed, Dandelion, Hawthorn, Garlic, Horseradish, Kelp, Parsley, Plantain, Papaya, Raspberry, Rosehips, Shepherds Purse, Yellow Dock.

The Safest Essential Oils For Animal Use

Supplement To The Natural Remedies For Animal Series

Though this is not specifically for goats these oils have been safely used in animals. I haven't altered this section but left it so you can get some ideas from the formulas used and maybe adapt them to you're your own purposes.

Extreme care must be taken using the Essential Oils on animals. The ones mentioned in these pages seem to be the safest if used in a low dose which is a quarter of what you would use on a human and even this would be too high if used on a mouse so really think about what you are doing and always use a little test dose to check for sensitivity.

Danger – Do not use on **birds** and **cats** as there metabolism cannot handle Essential oils and death will be the most likely result, this includes Eucalyptus and Tea Tree oil.

How Oils Work

Essential Oils work by entering the blood stream via the pores of the skin so the biggest action is on the area applied followed by a systemic action via the blood. The liver is the main blood filter and detoxifier of the body so the liver is responsible for breaking down any drug or blood borne foreigner so with the Essential Oils there is always the chance that if the dose is too high or the application is to frequent the liver may be damaged. Never forget that oils are highly concentrated products. A good example is a budgie, you clipped the wings and one is now bleeding so you put Tea Tree oil on it. Imagine the size of one drop of oil now imagine the size of a Budgies liver and it's fairly obvious what's going to happen.

Below are given the cautions for using oils on dogs, follow these cautions on all animals in general. Most information for these pages was sourced from Kristen Leigh Bells book Holistic Aromatherapy For Animals and Catharine Birds book A Healthy Horse The Natural Way.

Essential Oil Blends

Soothing Skin Essential Oil Blend

15ml base oil of hazel nut or sweet almond oil
2 drops Geranium
6 drops Rosewood
6 drops Lavender
1 drop Roman Chamomile
2 drops Carrot Seed

Combine all ingredients, shake and store in a dark glass bottle. Use 2 to 4 drops of this blend to spot treat small areas of skin.

Mange Treatment Blend

15ml base oil of hazel nut or sweet almond oil
5 drops Lavender

7 drops Niaouli
1 drop Helichrysum
2 drops Sweet Marjoram
After bathing the dog 2 to 4 drops of the blend should be applied to the affected areas twice a day for at least 2 weeks. Observe for a week and repeat if necessary. Try to prevent the dog from licking the area.

Tick Bite Forula
15ml base oil of hazel nut or sweet almond oil
5 drops Thyme Thujanol
3 drops Hyssop Decumbens
8 drops Lavender
For use on bites or immediately after the tick is removed to help prevent infection, reduce redness and inflammation and possibly prevent Lymes disease.

Fresh Breath Oil Blend
5ml base oil of hazel nut or sweet almond oil
6 drops Cardamom
4 drops Coriander Seed
6 drops Peppermint
1 to 3 drops inside of the dog's mouth.

Calm Dog Blend
15ml base oil of hazel nut or sweet almond oil
3 drops Valerian
2 drops Vetiver
4 drops Petitgrain
3 drops Sweet Marjoram

2 drops Sweet Orange
The calming effect ranges from taking the edge off to soothing the dog. Dose is 1 to 6 drops depending on the size of the dog.

Fear or Seperation Anxiety
15ml base oil of hazel nut or sweet almond oil
1 drop Neroli
2 drops Sweet Bazil
4 drops Bergamot
6 drops Petitgrain
1 drop Ylang Ylang
Dose is 1 to 6 drops depending on size of dog.

Flea Free Blend
15ml base oil of hazel nut or sweet almond oil
4 drops Clary Sage
1 drop Citronella
7 drops Peppermint
3 drops Lemon
Store in dark glass bottle. 2 to 4 drops to the neck, chest, legs and tail base of the dog.

Tick Free Blend
15ml base oil of hazel nut or sweet almond oil
2 drops Geranium
2 drops Rosewood
3 drops Lavender
2 drops Myrhh
2 drops Opoponax
1 drop Bay Leaf

Store in dark glass bottle. 2 to 4 drops to the neck, chest, legs and tail base of the dog.

Increasing The Appetite
15ml base oil of hazel nut or sweet almond oil

2 drops Sweet Orange

2 drops Lemon

2 drops Grapefruit

2 drops Lime

2 drops Bergamot

For old and sick dogs this is a gentle appetite stimulant. 2 to 6 drops of the final blend to the neck and chest of the dog gently rubbed in. Repeat as needed up to 6 times per day.

Immune Boosting Blend
15ml base oil of hazel nut or sweet almond oil

2 drops Bay Laurel

2 drops Ravensare

2 drops Palmarosa

2 drops Eucalyptus

2 drops Niaouli

2 drops Coriander Seed

2 drops Thyme Thujanol

2 to 4 drops daily via massage to neck and chest.

Colds and Congestion
15ml base oil of hazel nut or sweet almond oil

5 drops Eucalyptus

5 drops Myrhh

5 drops Ravensare

For relieving nasal congestion or cold symptoms in dogs. 1 to 6 drops rubbed into neck or chest.

Fatigue Blend
15ml base oil of hazel nut or sweet almond oil
7 drops Rosemary
6 drops Tangerine
3 drops Ylang Ylang
Balancing and revitalizing for dogs that are suffering from fatigue and malaise.
2 to 4 drops daily via massage to neck and chest.

Flatulence Blend
15ml base oil of hazel nut or sweet almond oil
3 drops Caraway
3 drops Cardamom
3 drops Cinnamon
3 drops Nutmeg
3 drops Tangerine
1 to 2 drops placed on your dog's food and then 1 or 2 drops given after eating. Many dogs enjoy the taste of this spicy blend and will lick it off your hand. The spice oils of this blend are commonly found in food flavorings so digestion is regarded as safe.

Joint Rub Blend
15ml base oil of hazel nut or sweet almond oil
3 drops Black Pepper
4 drops Peppermint
3 drops Speramint
4 drops Juniper Berry

Good for muscle soreness, arthritis, hip dysplasia and sprains. Use 2 to 4 drops of the blend and try to rub in as close to the skin as possible. Do a patch test with this oil as it can be irritating. Patch tests can be done with drop of blend in the arm pit.

Motion Sickness Blend
15ml base oil of hazel nut or sweet almond oil
7 drops Ginger
8 drops Peppermint
Give 3 drops in the mouth

Labor Ease Blend
15ml base oil of hazel nut or sweet almond oil
6 drops Clary Sage
1 drop Neroli
5 drops Petitgrain
2 drops Lavender
1 drop Roman Chamomile
Calming and balancing blend, can be applied to the fur of the neck or chest or 1 to 4 drops can be rubbed in the belly.

Oils For Horses

The safest way to use Essential Oils on your horse are external massage and inhalation. When inhaled the Oil addresses the horses emotional states and stored memories as well as entering the body and having an effect with the most obvious here being Eucalyptus which acts as a bronchodilator (illegal for competition horses in some parts of the US). **Use blends in the same strengths as mentioned in dogs don't go over 2% oil in a blend. Only apply the blends to the affected areas. You can copy some of the dog formulas or make your own using the list of oils.**

Essential Oils For Animal Use
The Essential Oils below are fairly safe for Animal Use

Basil (Sweet) - Helpful for restoring mental balance and clarity. For animals that are suffering nervousness or anxiety, dogs with separation anxiety. Use sparingly (PMC30%). **Horses** – Helps to release most muscle spasms. Used before a event it minimizes the amount of uric acid in the blood and other toxic wastes from exercise. A warming winter oil feeding the muscle fibers and stimulating the blood flow. It is a expectorant removing mucous from a clogged respiratory system when rubbed into the chest and inhaled. Rubbed into the abdomen it may help to relieve the pain and symptoms of colic. May irritate the skin in high doses and don't use in pregnancy.

Bay Leaf – Good for a hair and fur tonic, ticks don't like it, good deodorizer.

Actions – Ant microbial.

Bay Laurel – Used in blends for boosting the

immune system especially in dogs. Use only in small amounts in blends.

Bergamot – Combines toning, strengthening and balancing effects with soothing, relaxing and uplifting qualities. Useful for the treatment of fungal conditions such as dog ear infections due to yeast overgrowth. Use in small doses as it can cause photosensitization. **Horse** – Use full for treating any skin complaint especially folliculitis, flaking skin and wounds. Good for lice infections and bites, aids in the healing of any wounds and reduces scar formation. Has a stimulating effect on appetite. Be cautious when applying to the skin of a gray horse or to sensitive skin areas that will be exposed to the sun as this oil can cause photosensitization or pigment changes.

Black Pepper – Warming and circulatory stimulant qualities with low toxicity and irritation. Good for sore muscles, joint pains, arthritis and hip dysplasia. **Horse** – Gives tone to skeletal muscles and warms any winter chills. Dilates local blood vessels and improves local blood flow to the muscles warming the muscles from inside. Arthritic joints respond well to pepper and helps with pain management when used over a long period of time. Strengthens the nervous system. May antidote Homoeopathics.

Caraway Seed – Good for digestive problems, wind, poor appetite, indigestion and bad breath.

Cardamom – Digestive problems, bad breath. **Horse** – Good for treating digestive problems of a nervous origin. Encourages the flow of saliva and good for loss of appetite. It is warming when the body feels cold and useful for easing coughs and respiratory complaints. Highly antiviral and second only to Eucalyptus in that respect. For stallions you can use it as an aphrodisiac. May irritate some sensitive skins.

Carrot Seed – Valuable oil in the use of skin care, dry flaky skin that is sensitive to allergens and prone to infections. **Horses** – Strengthens the mucous membranes so is good for respiratory conditions. Useful for regenerating the skin after wounds or skin diseases and it antiseptic action will deal with minor infections. Has a toning hormone like action that will encourage conception and assist the infertile mare.

Cedarwood Atlas – Gentle stimulating oil that increases circulation and stimulates the release toxins. Good for the skin and fleas don't like it. **Horse** - Sores that are slow to heal, saddle sores, folliculitis etc. and dry flaky skin, encourage the re-growth of coat and adds shine. Has a tonic effect on the kidneys. Dries out excess phlegm and runny noses and removes excess mucous from the respiratory system when inhaled.

Chamomile German – Powerful skin soothing ant inflammatory. Burns, allergic reaction and all types of skin irritations can be quickly calmed with this oil. The oil has a deep blue color.

Chamomile Roman – Valuable for soothing the central nervous system and relieving cramps spasms and muscle pains. It also has analgesic effects which may be used for wounds. In humans this has traditionally been used for teething. **Horse** – The strong analgesic properties relieve dull muscular aches and stubborn spasms. It can also relieve overworked and inflamed muscles. Can be used as a wash to relieve the pain of inflames wounds. Good for calming difficult and unruly horses. Good for unmanageable mares when they cycle.

Cinnamon Leaf – Use the leaf not the bark as the leaf is gentler. Excellent digestive tonic and good for flatulent dogs and is a powerful anti-microbial.

Citronella – Well known insect repeller.

Clary Sage – Sedates the central nervous system, good for calming blends. **Horse** – Has a strong regenerative power where hair loss is involved. Useful on puffy joints caused by long periods of standing. Any swelling in the kidney area caused by strenuous work or sluggish kidney function. Calms underlying tension and soothes anxiety. Useful for a mare having trouble conceiving or nervous of the stallion. Don't use during pregnancy.

Coriander Seed – A toning balancing and strengthening oil that promotes and supports the digestion. It is also a circulatory stimulant and thus a good addition to blends for sore joints, muscles or arthritis.

Eucalyptus Radiata – A well-known remedy for congestion of the respiratory system. The oil has anti-viral, anti-inflammatory and expectorant effects. Can be a flea repellant. Antidotes Homoeopathic remedies. **Horse** – Eases muscular aches and pains caused by over exertion, relieves rheumatic and nerve pains. The anti-viral action is good for respiratory infections and it also soothes the inflammation and reduces excess mucous. Heals sores prone to pus formation. Can be irritating to sensitive skin.

Frankincense – Used to strengthen a weakened immune system and is a good choice for any blend for a sick or elderly animal that needs a systemic boost. Can be used for skin aliments due to its anti-inflammatory and anti-bacterial qualities. Horse – Eases shortness of breath and helps any respiratory problem. Rejuvenating especially for those recovering from a serious injury, tonic for the aging and can be used as a pick me up. Good for stubborn hard to heal wounds. Has the ability to dispel fear and anxiety. Don't use during pregnancy.

Geranium – Has tonic and strong anti-fungal actions, suitable in the use of prevention and treatment of fungal ear infections. Also can be used in tick repellant formulas. **Horse** – Gentle analgesic, has diuretic properties and a tonic action on the liver and kidneys. Balance hormones and emotions so is good for erratic mood swings.

Ginger – Good for the digestive and circulatory systems. Used for motion sickness, sprains, strains and arthritis. **Horse** – Good for conditions caused by cold and dampness. Stimulates circulation to cold joints and is analgesic relieving arthritic and rheumatic pain, muscle spasms and sprains. Is a appetite stimulant and can relieve travel sickness. Careful on sensitive skins.

Grapefruit – Used for calming, deodorizing and also repelling insects particularly fleas. Has a tonic effect on skin, hair and tissues. Useful for animals with imbalanced sebum production. **Horse** – Gentle effective lymphatic stimulant that nourishes cells while removing toxins. Tonic to the liver. Careful on sensitive skins.

Helichrysum - Actions – Analgesic, anti-inflammatory, regenerative, good for the skin.

Hyssop Decumbens – Different from the normal hyssop. This one is a antiviral and antibacterial and anti-depressant. The oil is also nontoxic and irritating.

Juniper Berry – Stimulating to the circulatory system and good for use in blends used for arthritis and pain. Helpful for balancing oily skin and for acne, eczema and hair loss. **Horse** - Helps stimulate kidney function and this in turn helps to remove metabolic wastes. Don't use during pregnancy.

Labdunum – This oil is antibacterial and astringent. Used for wounds.

Lavender - Antibacterial, antipruritic (anti-itch), powerful regenerative properties. The oil acts as a sedative on the central nervous system. **Horse** – Is cell regenerating and hastens the healing process. Sedates and soothes any wound or emotion. Helps to dispel gas and eases muscle tightness.

Lemon – Calming, strong antibacterial, deodorizer. **Horse** – Stimulates the body to excrete toxins and wastes via the skin, gently astringent and encourages the movement and release of excess toxins. Supports the liver and kidneys. In the cold season gently addresses runny watery respiratory problems and boosts the immune system. For older horses it can be added to rheumatic blends.

Lemon Grass - Antiviral and has a calming effect. **Horse** – Relieves pain in aching muscles and makes the muscles supple. Careful on sensitive skin and around wounds.

Mandarin Green – Good for calming fear, anxiety or stress. **Horse** – Nourishes the peripheral circulation feeding any extremity that suffers from poor circulation. Helps with muscle spasms.

Marjoram – Calming, spasmolytic, strong antibacterial, bacterial infections, wound care and insect repelling.
Meant to be good for calming over amorous male dogs. **Horse** – Warms cold aching joints, relieves muscle spasms and draws bruising to the surface. Helps with the aches and pain of arthritis and swollen joints in old horses. Can help with travel sickness.

Myrrh – Anti-inflammatory, anti-viral, good for puppy teething, treating irritated or inflamed skin conditions or for adding to immune boosting blends. Good for repelling ticks. **Horse** – Its antiseptic action is useful for deep seated respiratory conditions when inhaled. Can be used in a compress to treat boils, chapped or weeping skin conditions and fungal conditions like ringworm. Has a stimulating toning action on the mares reproductive system. Use only short term and not during pregnancy.

Neroli – Calming, stress reduction, anxiety, used for blend for female dogs in labor to ease pain and stress.

Niaouli – Anti histamine, antibacterial, good for allergies manifesting on the skin as well as first aid. Use for cleaning and for preventing ear infections in dogs.

Nutmeg – Canine flatulence, reduces gas production and aids in indigestion and nausea. Stimulating to the circulatory system.

Sweet Orange – Calming, deodorizing, flea repellant, may help in excess sebum production of the skin.

Palmarosa – Antibacterial, antiviral. **Horse** – Helpful when the body is over heated, encourages cellular regeneration and aid hydration by encouraging the flow of fluids throughout the body. Good for stiff joints and aching back.

Patchouli – Gentle circulatory stimulant for the skin and coat and also acts as a insect repellant. **Horse** – Tissue regenerator that aids in the healing of wounds, may address old scar tissue if applied regularly. Used for treating sores that contain heat a compress will cool the wound and help heal. Helps the skin regain its elasticity. Has diuretic properties.

Peppermint – Stimulates circulation, analgesic,

sprains, strains, arthritis, repels fleas, flies, mossies' , itching, car sickness. **Horse** – Peppermint has a cooling and analgesic action on heated local injuries. Can burn sensitive skins. Antidotes Homoeopathics.

Ravensare – Anti viral and antibacterial. For animals with compromised immune systems or for young dogs that are prone to infections.

Rose – Stabilizing to the central nervous system, has a gentle tonifying effect to the skin good for adding to blends for itchy or irritated skin.

Rosemary – The oil is mucolytic acting as a expectorant and also aids in cell regeneration. May help in promoting and maintaining hair growth. **Horse** – Stimulates both the mental and physical body into action, can relieve pain without sedating.

Rosewood – The oil has antiviral and antibacterial properties and ticks are repelled by the scent of it. Good for skin conditions.

Spearmint – Similar actions to peppermint, repels fleas and other insects stimulates circulation to the area it is used.

Spikenarde – Calming and grounding, rejuvenating and regenerating to the skin, good for dogs with skin problems, has a similar range of action as valerian.

Thyme Linalol – Antibacterial, anti-fungal, good for skin problems and not as harsh as thyme.

Thyme Thujanol – Has all the benefits of the above thyme as well as being a immune system stimulant and live detoxifier. Can be used in the prevention of lymes disease applied immediately after a tick bite.

Valerian – Calming and grounding, good for dogs with separation anxiety or who are fearful of loud noises, storms, fireworks or new situations. Good as a tonic for the nervous system.

Vetiver – Used in blends for calming, circulatory tonic and strengthens the immune system. **Horse** – Used to treat aches and pains and is a tonic for most body systems. Used for debilitated and distressed horses.

Ylang Ylang – Deeply calming, used in fatigue blends. **Horses** – Commonly used as a aphrodisiac, has an affinity for the adrenal glands.

Notes

Notes

Notes

Notes

Notes

Notes

www.ingramcontent.com/pod-product-compliance
Lightning Source LLC
Chambersburg PA
CBHW071406170526
45165CB00001B/190